ENERGETIC
PREGNANCY

ENERGETIC PREGNANCY

A guide to
achieving balance, vitality, & wellbeing
from conception to birth & beyond

ELIZABETH DAVIS

Photographs by Suzanne Arms Wimberley

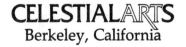
CELESTIALARTS
Berkeley, California

CELESTIAL ARTS
P.O. Box 7327
Berkeley, California 94707

Photographs © 1988 by Suzanne Arms Wimberley
Cover design by Ken Scott
Text design by Paul Reed & Nancy Austin
Typography by HMS Typography, Inc.
Centerfold illustrations © by Linda Harrison

LIBRARY OF CONGRESS
Library of Congress Cataloging in Publication Data

Davis, Elizabeth, 1950–
   Energetic pregnancy / by Elizabeth Davis.
     p.   cm.
   Includes index.
   ISBN 0-89087-522-7
   1. Pregnancy.   2. Obstetrics—Popular works.   I. Title.
   RG525.D525 1988   88-2978
   618.2′4—dc19   CIP

First Printing, 1988

1 2 3 4 5 – 92 91 90 89 88

Manufactured in the United States of America

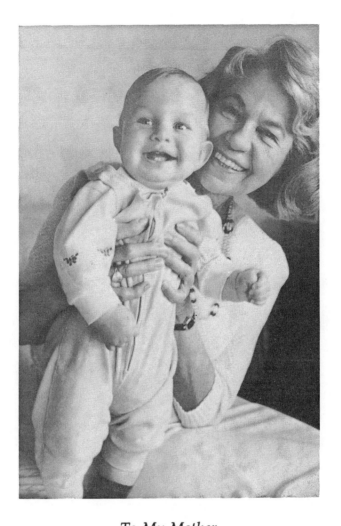

To My Mother
Marian Drake
One of a long line of liberated women
Who nevertheless believed
In the beauty and value
Of family

Contents

Acknowledgments

Deepest thanks to Jean Jones Burke, once my student and later my midwifery partner, for sharing insights on the psychology of women basic to this work. You have been a wonderful and trustworthy friend, a fine caregiver and facilitator! (Jean is a student of Da Free John.)

Special thanks to Suzanne Arms Wimberley, for contributing her lovely photographs and unique perspective to this project. Suzanne, you are an inspiration!

And to Linda Harrison, deep appreciation for the special touch of love and respect with which you portray pregnant women.

To Rose Dance, thanks for the encouragement and your excellent job of word processing the manuscript.

And to all the fine members of the Celestial Arts team, David Hinds, Paul Reed, Nancy Austin, Maryann Anderson, and Dayna Macy, my continuing appreciation for a job well done. Thank you!

Preface

I have been a midwife for almost ten years now, and gradually I've come to believe that my most important function in caregiving is to help a woman achieve a dynamic balance in her life. So many women are overwhelmed in pregnancy, struggling to sift through recommendations on nutrition, exercise and mental preparation with no idea of where to begin. This is because the starting point is different for everyone. By taking a complete physical history and assessing emotional wellbeing and mental attitude, I can size up a woman's areas of strength and weakness and assist her in focusing on aspects of herself that need attention. As she sets her priorities straight, she feels in control again.

My main reason for writing this book is to enable you, the expectant mother, to do this on your own, for yourself. Many of you may not have the benefit of individualized care and attention in pregnancy, and need some help sorting out essential preparation from routine advice, worthwhile activities from busywork.

With this sorting comes focus, a feeling of ease and relaxation as energies are no longer scattered or frantic. This is wholeness, your key to good health and the secret to an energetic pregnancy!

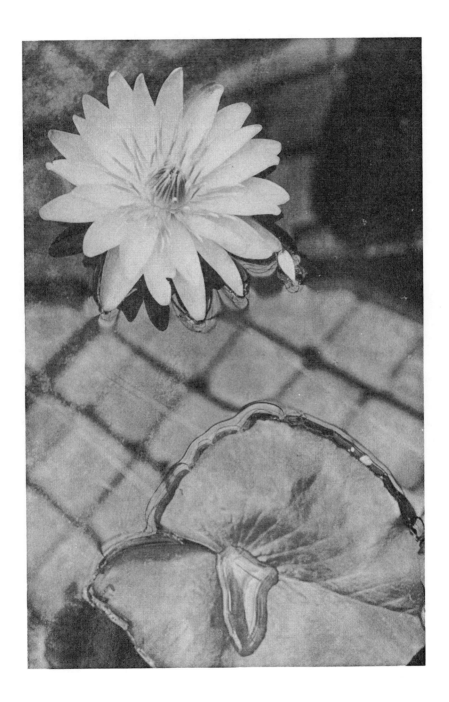

Chapter 1

Sources of Energy

An energetic pregnancy is surely something that every expectant mother desires. Especially today, when a woman must juggle career, relationships and personal interests with the demands of being pregnant. This is a tall order at best, and to make matters worse there is a veritable overrun of information on the ideal diet, optimal exercise and perfect mental attitude. It's no wonder that many pregnant women throw up their hands and wonder, "What about *me*? Don't I have any say in the matter? Don't I count anymore?"

Yes, there is another way, a more personalized path to follow. Intuition can figure mightily, rather than being drowned out by the advice and recommendations of others. Pregnancy can be a time of personal (not just fetal) growth and a precious, heightened phase in a woman's life. The key is personal balance; bringing your physical, emotional, mental and social sides into harmonious function. If you succeed at this, your day-to-day tasks and responsibilities will fall naturally into place.

However, you may have noticed that society has a somewhat different agenda. All too often, pregnant women are made to feel fragile, delicate or temporarily out-of-service; they are discouraged from active sports or intense lovemaking. Physicians may play a paternalistic role, coddling and protective, "Don't worry dear, I'll take care of everything." The concept of pregnant woman as passive vessel extends to birth practices as well; women are still expected to labor and give birth lying flat on their backs (the most uncomfortable and unnatural of positions) and to remain quiet throughout (although grunting and groaning are often involuntary). Just consider the terminology used to refer to the due date: EDC, or expected date of *confinement!*

On the other hand we have the opposite extreme, which might best be termed the "Amazon concept." This has many variations but all feature the expectant mother as essentially unchanged by her pregnancy, working right up to the first labor pain and resuming full activity immediately after giving birth. Proponents of this view claim it is rooted in primitive culture, where the mother at work in the fields supposedly squatted and birthed, swaddled her baby about her and continued on as though nothing had happened, or else wrapped up her newborn and jumped back on her horse! Contrary to popular belief, this is not the normal way among indigenous populations; instead, most observe a six-week period called lying-in wherein the new mother is completely cared for and protected from outside influences. This is true for the native cultures of Central America, Australia and Southeast Asia, to name a few. In fact, the transitional and somewhat precarious nature of the postpartum period is so well appreciated in the Phillippines that if the mother dies within the first forty days after giving birth, it is believed that her soul will automatically go to heaven (after that, she's on her own!)

Basic components of postpartum care in these cultures are seclusion, bedrest, good food and plenty of warmth. The latter is considered especially critical; often a fire is built either under the bed or very nearby and there is ritual regarding how the wood is cut, the fire laid, etc. The heat allows the mother to be nude, which promotes skin-to-skin contact with her infant and aids the bonding process. It is also said to reduce afterpains and blood loss, tone up the abdomen and promote easy lactation. Total nurturing allows for spontaneous sleep, nursing and interaction with the baby.

Quite probably, it was primitive cultures undergoing a threat to survival that found it necessary to bring new mothers immediately back into the work force. To do so runs contrary to nature, as the hormones that induce breastfeeding and restore the uterus to its normal size are severely inhibited by any release of adrenalin. Clearly, the "Amazon concept" is mostly myth.

Faced with these extremes, and bereft of any cultural traditions that support the natural course of childbearing, how are we to create our own middle ground? We can devise our own health-promoting rituals, and share them with other women of like mind. But first we must understand the basic phases of pregnancy and how they fit together. And we must face the fact that pregnancy causes definite physiological changes in us which require adjustments. For example, the hormone progesterone dilates and softens blood vessels, leading to various circulatory disturbances. Thus the tendency of pregnant women to feel faint or dizzy is not emotionally induced, nor is the common complaint of breathlessness: both are due to increased demands for oxygen. It is critical to appreciate these physical changes so we don't feel victim to them and can therefore enlighten distressed family and friends if necessary.

Beyond a doubt, one of the most critical keys to a spontaneous and healthful pregnancy is *adaptation*. There is a passage from a Chinese book of wisdom that says it perfectly, "No situation can become favorable until one ceases to wear oneself out with mistaken resistance." Unfortunately it is typical of our culture to find such a path threatening in its simplicity. Deep down, we know such adaptation requires more than a little self-discipline, patience and acceptance, quite the opposite of our usual ways of self-indulgence and instant gratification. Above and beyond all else, we want to have fun! To this end, we're more inclined to look for some fad or technique, some food or supplement to "give us energy" than to the metaphysical shape we're in. *This*

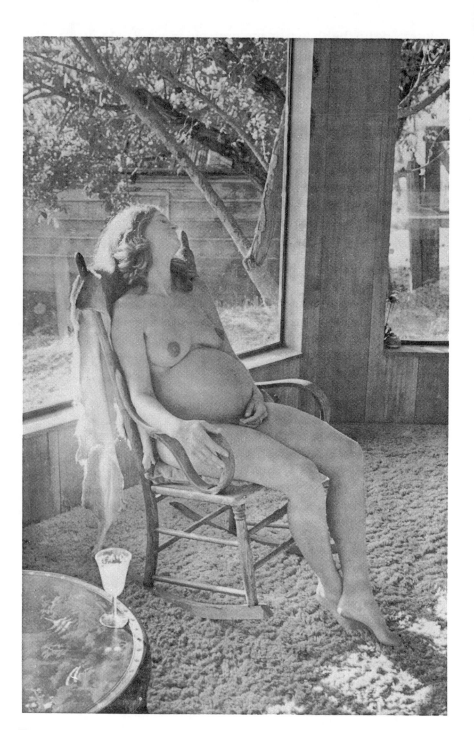

is because we perceive energy as coming from an outside source, rather than from inside ourselves. This is an essentially masculine orientation to life, and our society caters to it. Advertising persuades us that we cannot be complete without adding unto ourselves, be it the right diet drink, life insurance policy, hamburger or hair color. And when we need "a lift," what do we go for? A candy bar, a richer cup of coffee, better hair conditioner or a new car. *We are confusing energy with stimulation!* Stimulation is temporary, transitory; it keeps us coming back for more. And when the newness or thrill of a particular source wears off we go looking again, and never really settle into our own energy.

Fortunately, pregnancy provides a unique opportunity to settle in this way, as the hormones work to slow us down, heighten our sensitivities and make us more physically aware. The pregnant body definitely has an order, rhythm and logic all its own; ask any woman in her first trimester! Understanding and *working with* this order will allow a naturally energetic feeling to ensue.

Don't worry, this doesn't have to be boring! Replace any puritanical notions of self-discipline with images of playful, sensual attunement. You can use your feminine sensibilities, your dreams, fantasies and intuitions to develop these for yourself.

And here is where the fine tuning comes in. Each of us is a complex mosaic of attributes, with definite strengths and weaknesses. What's more, appropriate techniques of preparation vary from person to person, or to rephrase an old adage, "One woman's meat is another woman's poison." A bit of self analysis, using the guidelines and information presented in this book, will help you figure out where you need some work or improvement and how best to allocate your resources.

This will enable you to conserve energy, rather than frittering it away unnecessarily. For example, a woman with a long standing focus on nutrition, whose initial diet analysis checks out well, need not revamp herself in this area where she is already strong. Neither should a woman accustomed to a certain type or level of physical activity stop suddenly when she becomes pregnant. This principle may seem obvious and easy to apply, but often we are blind to our own assets and liabilities. Again, the case histories and quizzes in the coming chapters will help you figure out where you stand.

In my work as a midwife, I've had ample opportunity to observe the importance of personal balance when labor finally comes around. Labor requires all-systems-go; for most women it takes everything they've got (and then some). It works a woman *on all levels;* any area that has been blocked or neglected in pregnancy is bound to be revealed and may cause some serious obstacles to progress.

Not only is balance crucial in terms of birthing, but essential to happy and successful parenting. You will enjoy your role as mother much more if you are unafraid and ready to engage in various types of activities with your child. It pays to remember, and to remind yourself from time to time that pregnancy is not just preparation for birth, but for becoming a parent.

Keep in mind that the term balance as I use it here refers not to a static (and therefore precarious) state, but to a dynamic flow of vital energies ultimately contributing to overall growth. It depends on self-awareness; your willingness to pay attention to personal needs and take a few chances for self development.

Chapter 2

The Cyclical Nature of Pregnancy and Birth

For many women, the news of pregnancy is accompanied by a strange sense of terror. Not to say that there isn't happiness and elation too, but a feeling of fear is not uncommon. Even if the whole thing has been carefully planned, the reality of *actually being pregnant* is quite different from the fantasy. What is it about pregnancy that is so unnerving, that can reduce an otherwise strong and rational woman to quivering anxiety and apprehension?

I'll never forget the moment I got the test results on my last pregnancy. I had wanted another baby for a number of years and yet, when the blue dot appeared in the test container that signaled "positive," I felt shaken to the core. Thrilled and exhilarated but shaken nonetheless! I felt my reality slipping, shifting to another dimension. Not only was my body starting to change, but I knew that my primary relationships, career, lifestyle and finances would soon be affected in ways I could barely imagine. But beyond all else I felt a fear of the unknown, of losing control.

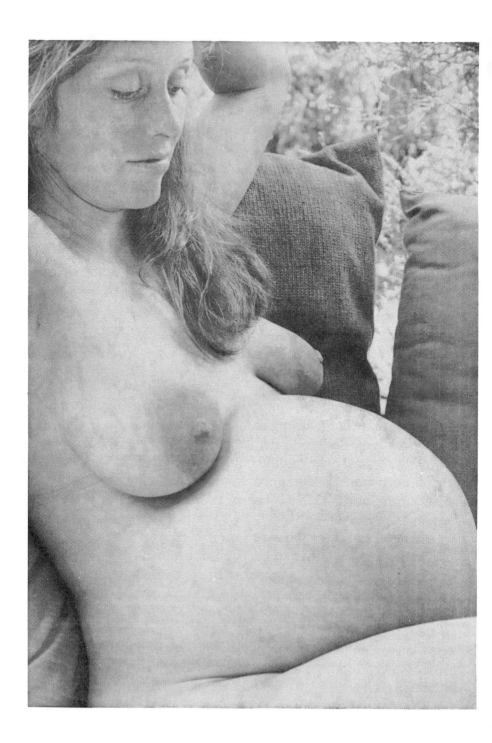

It was as though I was barreling full-throttle toward some destination that could not be foreseen.

Although our culture does little to acknowledge the fact, childbirth is a *transitional* experience, a bridge from one chapter of existence to another from whence one emerges a changed being. As such, birth deeply affects the psyche and evokes our most primal and intense emotions. It is almost impossible to put into words the transformation of becoming a parent, the way you feel when you see your baby for the first time. And as a veteran of three totally different birth experiences (and a mother of three completely different children) I can attest with utter certainty that it's never twice the same; you never "get it down."

Yet, even though birth is characterized by powerful and intensified energy, it is not random or chaotic in unfolding. Whether labor moves slowly or quickly, it follows a certain pattern. Likewise, the whole of pregnancy has definite stages with certain characteristics. From conception to postpartum, the phases fit together like pieces of a puzzle. In fact, the entire process is cyclical in nature. One returns full-circle to the starting point (the nonpregnant self) and begins anew as a parent.

The first trimester is a time of adjustment, an emotional phase of feeling things through. Women who work may feel inconvenienced by the erratic demands of their appetites or unpredictable needs for rest. And those who have spent many years putting themselves "in order" may be quite distressed by moodswings and personality changes, which further disrupt routine. In order to enjoy and be responsive to all this, you must be patient enough to explore and unfold new ways of being. In a nutshell, this is a time to tune into your inner voice and intuition as never before. The more your body changes, the more any struggle to maintain the status quo will be doomed to failure. Make the sacrifice to union with your baby, and activate deeper levels of understanding. The main message of the early months is to let go of outmoded concepts and let yourself *grow!*

Thus you pave the way for a balanced and integrated midpregnancy. As your body becomes adjusted and you move past the hormonal upsets of nausea and fatigue, you will find new vitality. The baby begins to make itself known to you with turns, kicks and subtle communication. All the world can see that you are pregnant and it's a pleasure, with new routines of eating, rest and activity tried and true. This is a time of emotional equilibrium, a time for sharing with other pregnant women and with your mate and closest friends, who may have wondered if you were ever going to even-out again!

And then the wheel turns again, the balance shifts and the birth is felt to be impending. The last trimester is a time of rapid growth for the baby to the point where it feels cramped and confined, and you will feel correspondingly overwhelmed and overburdened. Lost sleep, fatigue, indigestion and awkwardness with intercourse can be seen as major inconveniences, or accepted as stimuli to develop patience and the ability to abide disruption of your own needs for the sake of the baby. Emotions are often uncontrollable at this time; many women feel filled to overflowing and find themselves weeping daily. But this is good, for the yielding up of every last bit of resistance makes the labor process easier.

As labor begins, pregnancy is ending. Harking back to the first trimester, the early phase of labor is a period of mixed emotions. There is nostalgia for pregnancy passing away, and some last-minute anxiety. But these feelings quickly give way to elation, optimism and a burst of energy. Let your emotions flow freely, but resist any impulse to busy yourself or you might get too tired for the hard work to come. If labor begins at night it's wise to rest as long as possible; if it begins during the day, be satisfied with light chores or calming activities like a walk outdoors.

As contractions become strong and compelling, the excitement and adjustment of early labor give way to reckoning. Many women will take their time in reaching this point, coming up to it and backing off several times before finally going ahead. This is fine, as long as the contractions are still of variable intensity. But if your body is attempting to shift gears and move ahead into active labor and you persist in working against it, you will exhaust

Psychological Changes in Pregnancy
(from Helen Varney's *Nurse Midwifery*)

The First Trimester: Period of Adjustment
(the woman focuses on herself)

- She validates the pregnancy over and over, by noting each and every body change
- Even if she has planned the pregnancy, she may feel ambivalent (80% of women have feelings of anxiety, depression, disappointment or unhappiness)
- Perceives herself and the baby as one

The Second Trimester: Period of Radiant Health
(the woman focuses on the baby)

Before feeling movement:
- She may relive her relationship with her mother, analyzing positive and negative aspects
- She develops her own definition of mothering and evolves from care receiver to caregiver

After feeling movement:
- She tends to let go of old friendships and aspects of her former role as a non-parent; may experience grief in doing so
- If she already has children, may disengage and redefine ties within the family
- Perceives the baby as a separate individual

The Third Trimester: Period of Watchful Waiting
(the woman focuses on the birth)

- She engages in active preparation, takes birth classes, organizes the baby's room, etc.
- Is protective of the baby and may avoid crowds or stressful situations
- Usually experiences grief for the pregnancy passing away
- Is increasingly uncomfortable and eager to give birth

yourself when you've barely begun. The keys to progress are *surrender and acceptance.* You'll need to find a somewhat comfortable position to settle into for a while, as you make your adjustment. Sitting cross-legged with arms, neck and shoulders relaxed is preferable to side-lying, which is often disorienting and does little to aid the baby's descent. Early labor is similar to the first months of pregnancy when you search for the best emotional and physical stance for getting on with it and find you must let go of old concepts; in this case, ideas of what labor is supposed to be like. With this release you become more receptive to your sensations, and as they intensify and increase so will dilation. Your breathing in labor will flow instinctively if you don't interfere with arbitrary, preconceived patterns.

At about six or seven centimeters of dilation the contractions become so strong that they require your total attention. As you concentrate on relaxation and keeping the pace with your breathing, you'll find that you begin to move along almost automatically. Characteristically, this is a time of peace for many women. One feels strained and stretched to the full, and one-pointed on giving way as fully as possible.

Your breathing may accelerate slightly, echoing the energy coursing through you. The rhythm of breathing and resting, breathing and resting is so continuous that it is almost hypnotic. As the contractions intensify, you'll find yourself sinking deeper and deeper between times into a very still and peaceful state (imperative for recuperation). This is the point of discovering, at last, that labor is much bigger than you are. Many women worry while pregnant that they'll never be able to handle hours of painful sensation, with no chance to take a time-out. The truth is that labor alters normal, every-day reality so greatly that time ceases to exist. In addition, the body releases narcotic-like substances called endorphins, which considerably raise the pain threshold. Consequently a woman can be frightened and crying at three or four centimeters of dilation and smiling and relaxed at eight. A common feeling at this stage is that contractions rise like the wind and sweep through you, blowing you open and carrying you to the outer reaches where you rest, at one with the source. And this is no poetic exaggeration! This blissful state rejuvenates a woman and helps her find the courage to go on.

Along with the cyclical movement of each contraction, the overall cycle of labor is moving along its way. The entire first stage is really a process of ego dissolution, and many women find it akin to what they imagine dying to be like. The atmosphere in the birthing room at this time is usually one of profound peace. There is quiet, broken only by the sound of the mother's breathing and the gentle encouragement of friends and attendants, then quiet again. Occasionally it is necessary to reposition the mother for comfort or to help the baby move down, but her resting periods should always be respected and interrupted as little as possible.

And then everything changes; labor reaches a peak and a turning point. We call this stage "transition." Envisioning the birth process as a circle, transition marks the beginning of the return.

Transition is confusing because the body is doing two things at once; completing the dilation (with the most intense contractions thus far) and simultaneously beginning the downward efforts of expulsion. Along with the need for complete passive cooperation you feel unsettling urges to do something, even though what to do may not yet be clear! Almost every woman feels restless at this point and expressions of frustration are common, be they emotional outbursts or abrupt physical movements. Know that *transition means change*; since you can't resist conflicting urges chaos will reign for a while. Some women have just moments of transition, but if the baby is posterior and must accomplish a long rotation, transition may last for several hours. If this is your situation the only thing to do is persevere and try to accept the awkwardness. In essence, transition calls you back into your body and moves you on to the active work of pushing. Making moaning sounds and rocking your body in a sensual way can help you reckon with this change. The sensation level is outrageous; I recall yelling out during my daughter's birth at the height of transition, "I can't *do* this anymore!" but suddenly felt her head slip down in my vagina and (grunt, squeeze, umm) I was anchored in the new work of pushing.

The second stage of labor is the home stretch. Though if the baby's head has not descended sufficiently to stimulate the pushing urge, you may linger initially in this phase without much direction. The feeling of limbo can be disconcerting, but is often nature's way of giving you a rest after an arduous first stage. Women who have borne children and have great flexibility in their tissues may on the other hand move immediately into full-bodied pushing, with no chance to ease in emotionally. In any event, once the baby's head is low and true bearing down urges do ensue, their phenomenal power and your ability to cooperate will most likely astound and thrill you. Cooperation *is* the key; you should breathe into contractions as long as comfortably possible and bear down according to the strength of your impulse. If the contraction is very strong you will feel your ribs and diaphragm fix in place automatically, and have only to catch a breath and follow through with the involuntary squeeze. If the next is more mild, ease into it with your breathing and press down as it peaks, perhaps several small presses rather than one sustained. Second stage is like a dance, or like sensitive love-making with its ebb and flow. Getting into this responsive rhythm and feeling the incredible stimulation of the baby's head on sensitive vaginal tissues builds up an erotically changed energy much like the excitement preceding orgasm. It's very important to keep your mouth loose (there is a neuro-muscular association between mouth and vagina) and to let free any sounds that may well up inside you. Keeping the pitch of your voice low helps you open up and give in to the pressure.

Second stage contractions build in intensity, and the resting phase has the same out-of-body quality as the end of first stage. But as long as there is no undue exertion, your alertness is maintained by the charge and excitement of anticipation. You build an internal focus, which prepares you for the sensitive work of easing the baby out. As delivery approaches you begin to sense when to bear down, when to ease up and when to hold a stretch,

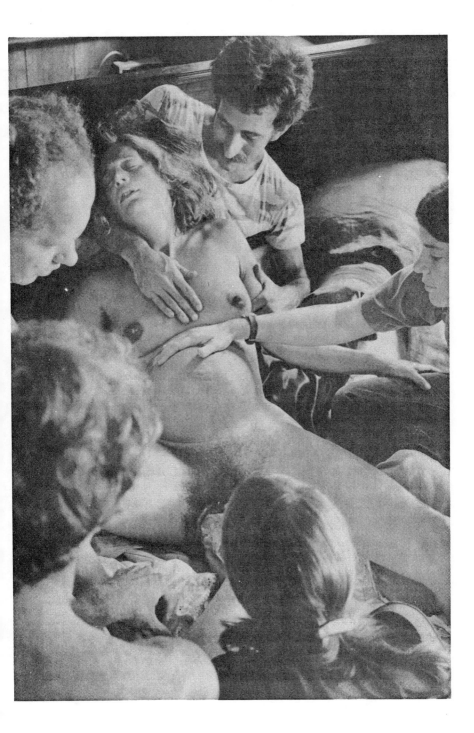

thus greatly reducing your likelihood of tearing. Reaching down to touch the baby's head helps you connect the boundless realm of sensation with the material fact of your body. Looking in the mirror does the same thing.

The moments of actual delivery are probably the most intense moments in a woman's life. All your energy is poised, focused on the transition from inside to outside. When the head is ready to ease out and you are fully stretched, pant lightly and surrender completely by making yourself a wide open channel. This way you will be able to feel each part of the baby moving through you, your first intimate tracing of its form. As the baby slithers out you will feel great relief and ecstasy, and may also feel a fleeting sense of loss or emptiness just before you put your baby to breast (the end of one cycle, the beginning of another).

This experience of sheer joy and fulfillment is birth, and you are reborn in the bargain. When you hear that first cry, all that has been suspended, all the expectations of the long wait are allowed to rush forward. Hormones are triggered, the uterus clamps down and third stage begins. Grantly Dick-Read observed that third stage was like a mini-labor with mild contractions, transitional anxiety and physical focus as the placenta delivers. Then the process is really complete. Third stage is an anti-climax, a way for energy that has reached such intensity to unwind itself slowly. Think of the way a storm breaks, or of diminishing aftershocks following an earthquake. This is nature's way.

Many women experience a special sort of sleep right after delivery, several hours long and deeply therapeutic. (It is said that if this sleep is interrupted, sleep-hunger lasting for several days can result.) Ordinarily the entire family falls asleep together, and wakes feeling refreshed and very happy!

In the days that follow, the baby helps you find your way from the exalted state of birth back to the ordinary concerns of living. Despite fatigue and upsets to routine, your love for your newborn infuses responsibility with joy. This is the bonding period, a time of delicacy in establishing harmony together. You may find that the desire for privacy lingers: the baby comes before

Phases in the First Six Weeks Postpartum

(adapted from an old nursing text, author unknown)

Phase One: Taking In (Day 1–Day 3)

The new mother:

- Is passive-dependent overall; she is a *receiver.*

- Wants plenty of rest and sleep.

- Is *very* hungry, if in the hospital will find meals to be inadequate (friends/family should bring extra).

- Needs to review details of the birth with attendants in order to assimilate and go on.

Phase Two: Taking Hold (Day 4–Day 10)

The mother now:

- Becomes the initiator, the *producer.*

- Actively re-masters care of herself and gives directions to her family on how to assist her.

- Begins to organize care of the baby, once she feels some autonomy in caring for her own needs.

Phase Three: Taking Charge (11 Days–6 Weeks)

The mother continues:

- To test her capabilities, with increasing success.

- To experience postpartum fatigue, partly due to physical exhaustion but also to her own inner drive for excellence.

- To be hypercritical of herself, vulnerable and in need of ongoing support.

all else. Give yourself all the time in the world, be sensitive to your needs for all manner of nourishment and allow the birth atmosphere to dissolve slowly.

The first three months postpartum have been called the fourth trimester, because it takes about that long for you and your baby to get your rhythms in harmony. You are establishing breastfeeding and getting your body back, and your baby is adjusting on many levels to life on this planet. You can utilize all the lessons learned in giving birth as per patience, surrender and acceptance to enable you to endure interrupted sleep, emotional upheavals and other familial stresses. Just remember that ultimately, you had to find your own way and rely on yourself during labor, and so it is with mothering as well. After all, the baby is not some abstract, alien little being but *your own child*. By believing in your inherent connection and allowing for gradual coming together, you will probably find that by the time the fourth month rolls around, you and your baby will be ready to turn out to the world at large.

Chapter 3

Physical Changes: Cause and Effect

Getting used to being pregnant is not always easy. There are many physical changes; so much more involved than just growing a baby! The heart works harder, since your blood volume increases by nearly 50% (this is to insure that both you and your baby have adequate oxygen for your needs). The thyroid gland, which regulates growth and other body functions, grows 50% bigger in pregnancy. The overall rate of your metabolism drops at first (which probably accounts for the fatigue many women experience in early pregnancy) but then rises steadily until the baby comes. The skeleton undergoes changes too; as muscles and ligaments soften, the pelvis enlarges and the ribs flare out to allow for deeper respiration. The muscle coat of the vagina expands to allow for stretching during delivery, and the breasts enlarge and prepare for lactation.

By and large, these changes are due to the action of hormones. We all know from our menstrual cycles how intensely hormones can affect us, both physically and emotionally. Obviously the hormonal changes of pregnancy are more sweeping, and the emotional ups and downs they cause more exaggerated. The better we understand how these hormones work, the less we'll feel victim to their influences.

When it comes to common complaints during pregnancy, the hormone that's implicated time and again is *progesterone.* Be it heartburn, constipation or varicosities, elevated progesterone levels are usually at fault. But what *is* progesterone, where does it come from and why do we need more of it than usual while pregnant?

Progesterone is one of two star players in our monthly menstrual cycle; the other is estrogen, which we will discuss a little later. Around mid-cycle after ovulation has occurred, progesterone levels rise *temporarily* to produce a healthy uterine lining, just in case of conception. If fertilization of the egg does not occur, progesterone levels drop and the lining is shed as menstruation. But if conception does take place, levels of progesterone *stay high* to maintain the uterine environment so the ovum can implant. Progesterone further serves to reduce uterine muscle irritability, so that the uterus will retain its contents. At first progesterone is made by the ovaries, but soon after implantation the placenta takes over and begins producing it instead.

Take a look at illustration I, center insert. This will show you, at a glance, the effects of hormones on your pregnant body. Overall, progesterone has a relaxing effect on smooth muscle, which accounts for many of these conditions. As we consider these briefly one-by-one, I will suggest remedies that represent a synthesis of many sources. Skip through these sections if you wish and read only those that apply to you.

Let's consider CONSTIPATION first, a frequent first-trimester complaint. Progesterone softens the smooth muscles of the intestines so they slow down, which causes the bowels to back up a bit. On the other hand, because food spends additional time in the intestines, absorption of nutrients is better; in short, this is nature's way of seeing that you get the most from what you eat. Eventually your body adjusts (although in the last trimester the baby's head may pose a physical obstacle to moving your bowels easily).

You can try:

1) Fiber-rich foods, like bran cereal, raw vegetables, etc.

2) Plenty of water, 2-3 quarts daily.

3) Regular exercise, to stimulate circulation and keep the bowels moving.

4) In emergency, a cup of prune juice or a large bowl of bran cereal.

Avoid:

1) Laxative preparations, unless they are the bulk-forming variety such as Metamucil or Effersyllium. Over-the-counter medicines such as Ex-Lax may be harmful to your baby.

HEMORRHOIDS are also caused by the softening action of progesterone. In this case, it's the blood vessels supplying the anus which dilate and prolapse downward. This can happen early in pregnancy along with constipation, or later as the enlarged uterus puts pressure on the hemorrhoidal veins. Hemorrhoids can also develop during delivery with extreme bearing down.

You can try:

1) Avoiding constipation by using the measures suggested in the previous section.

2) Putting your feet up on a stool while having a bowel movement, to avoid straining.

3) Doing Kegels to promote circulation and venous return (blood flow back towards the heart from the rectal area).

4) Pads of witch hazel (like Tucks) to relieve pain and itching. You can keep these chilled in the refrigerator for better effect.

Avoid:

1) Hemorrhoidal medications in general. Preparation H has a local anesthetic which may be absorbed into your bloodstream and could cause harm to the baby.

VARICOSE VEINS are caused in the same way as hemorrhoids; in addition, the pressure of the baby's head late in pregnancy against major vessels leading into the legs may further impair circulation.

You can try:

1) Regular exercise. This is really important! Not just stop-and-go walking around the house, but exercise! Swimming is particularly helpful.

2) Wearing support hose. You may need to visit an undergarment specialty shop to find what you need. Pantyhose are quite uncomfortable; stockings are best. These can be rigged to a large size garter belt, worn high with garters fully extended. One of my clients attached her stockings to a sanitary belt worn low. Be on the lookout for new products or use your imagination, just be sure there is nothing tight across your belly or upper thighs.

3) Loose clothing on the legs; no knee-hi nylons or knee socks.

4) Putting your feet up, or better yet, lying down with your feet elevated for several short periods during the day.

5) Wearing low-heeled, *comfortable* shoes to reduce the stress on your legs.

6) Taking extra vitamin E. Try 600 units daily.

FREQUENT URINATION early in pregnancy is due to the softening of pelvic muscles so that the uterus falls forward against the bladder, causing pressure and a limited amount of room for urine. As the uterus enlarges and moves upward, the pressure is relieved. However, the problem may reoccur at the end of pregnancy when the baby's head is low in the pelvis.

You can try:

1) Drinking plenty of fluids early in the day and decreasing your intake at night, so you won't have to get up often.

Avoid:

1) Limiting fluid intake. This is dangerous for you and the baby.

DIZZINESS AND FAINTING are due to circulatory disturbances caused, once again, by progesterone. The dilation of major vessels causes blood to pool in the legs, which slows return to the heart. And as the uterus enlarges it may press against these vessels, which further compounds the problem.

You can try:

1) Getting up from resting positions slowly.

2) Moving more slowly in general. One of my clients had a fainting spell after running for a bus and plopping down abruptly in her seat.

3) Lying down when you do feel faint, so blood will flow to your head.

HEADACHE may also be caused by circulatory disturbances, or as a reaction to hormone changes. It is definitely more common in early pregnancy; in fact, if it occurs later in pregnancy and in conjunction with swelling of the face or visual disturbances, contact your care provider immediately to rule out preeclampsia.

You can try:

1) Applying a cold cloth to your forehead and the back of your neck.

2) Lying down, both to increase circulation and induce relaxation.

3) Having a friend massage your head, neck and shoulders.

4) Allowing yourself emotional release; say what you're feeling, get angry or cry if you need to.

5) Hot herb tea, such as chamomile or scullcap (or commercial blend for inducing sleep).

Avoid:

1) Taking medications if possible. Tylenol is preferable to aspirin, particularly in the last three months when the latter can cause internal bleeding.

HEARTBURN is caused by the softening action of progesterone on the valve which separates the stomach and esophagus, so that the acid contents of the stomach escape upwards through the valve. Since the esophagus has no protective coating like the stomach, the acids cause a burning sensation. The problem is compounded by slowed digestion, in that often the stomach is backed up or overfull. Generally heartburn is worse in the later months when the growing baby puts pressure on the stomach, and is particularly troublesome when the mother lies down and gravity no longer holds the stomach acids in their proper place.

You can try:

1) Several small meals spread throughout the day. Eat lightly in the evening.

2) Plenty of fluids, again, taken throughout the day.

3) Eating cheese, or sipping buttermilk when heartburn strikes.

4) Taking digestive enzymes, papain and bromelain (derived from papaya and pineapple). Keep a bottle at your bedside, and take as needed.

5) Sleeping with the head and shoulders elevated.

6) The butterfly exercise. Sit cross-legged, and raise your arms several times in rapid succession, each time letting your hands meet above your head.

7) Gelusil or Maalox, which will not harm the baby (take only in recommended quantities).

Avoid:

1) Bicarbonate of soda, or medications like Alka-Seltzer, Fiz-rin, Soda Mint, Eno or Rolaids, which all contain too much sodium. These can disrupt your metabolism in a way that is definitely dangerous for you and your baby.

NOSEBLEEDS AND BLEEDING GUMS are both caused by the softening and dilating of the blood vessels, compounded by pressure created by increased blood volume.

For both, you can try:

1) Vitamin E, 600 units a day, and vitamin C complex with bioflavinoids and rutin, 500 mg. daily.

For gums specifically, have your teeth cleaned during your pregnancy. Most dentists prefer to wait until the second trimester, as there is a risk that infectious material might enter the bloodstream and damage the fetus if still in the formative stage. However, progesterone exaggerates the susceptibility of your tissues to plaque so you should definitely have a cleaning at least once in pregnancy.

For nosebleeds specifically, avoid nosedrops, as they can harm the baby and do little good in the long run.

———————————

These are the major side effects of progesterone on pregnancy; there are others caused by different hormones. *Estrogen,* for example, is the other star player in your monthly cycle. Also produced by the ovaries, it causes the growth of the uterine lining (which progesterone maintains) and is responsible for breast growth, changes in the vagina and cervix, and uterine enlargement.

It is also primarily responsible for NAUSEA in the early months, although other hormones, like human chorionic gonadotrophin (HCG) may also be at fault. It is much more apt to occur when the stomach is empty (hence the term morning sickness) although it may also occur in the evening in response to cooking odors. It is reassuring to know that over 50% of pregnant women experience this to some degree. Although there has been speculation that nausea may indicate a toxic condition of the system, I think it is more likely a simple reaction to hormones. In fact, some authorities believe it to be a *good* sign, an indication that the pregnancy is a good "take" because hormone levels are so high. Whatever the cause, it is certainly unpleasant and disruptive of schedules! Should nausea ever give way to repeated episodes of vomiting, contact your care provider.

You can try:

1) Keeping your stomach full but not overfull, by eating/nibbling small portions throughout the day.

2) Increasing your protein intake.

3) Eating dry crackers or plain yogurt first thing in the morning.

4) Increased amounts of vitamin B6. For *many* women this is the solution! Try 50 mg. at bedtime and another 50 mg. mid-day.

5) Fresh air, favorite activities, pampering yourself.

6) Asking your mate to do the little things you know will make you feel comfortable, secure, loved. This is good practice for labor, parenting and the rest of your lives together.

Avoid:

1) Taking medications, even if your physician says they are safe. Remember Thalidomide, which doctors thought was safe until they found out otherwise, and more recently Bendectine, which was pulled from the market after being implicated in several cases of fetal deformity. *Be most cautious* in this regard, avoid any over-the-counter medications.

2) Greasy, fatty or highly spiced foods, coffee, black tea and processed sweets.

FATIGUE in pregnancy is also due to elevated estrogen levels, although the lowered metabolic rate caused by progesterone may also be at fault. And during the first few months when your body is forming the placenta and baby, tremendous energy and resources are required even though you don't appear to be doing anything! Let go of notions that need for sleep indicates laziness or loss of control. Your body is *hard at work;* allow it to function spontaneously and the latter part of your pregnancy will be healthier and easier for you.

During the final few weeks of pregnancy you may feel tired once again from carrying the extra weight of the baby, or from emotional fluctuations. Nevertheless, always remember that *fatigue is a sign from your body that you need rest.*

You can try:

1) Acceptance.

2) Taking short (or long, if your schedule permits) naps.

3) Going to bed earlier, like 9 pm. for instance!

4) Regular exercise. This will energize you and actually *reduce* fatigue.

Towards the end of pregnancy there are certain problems caused by the physical stresses of carrying a baby. Most of these are caused in part by hormones, but are mainly due to organ displacement or muscle and ligament strain (see illustrations II and III, center insert).

ANKLE EDEMA is largely due to the baby's head impinging on major blood vessels and impairing circulation. Often there is no lasting remedy until the baby is born. Part of nature's protective plan for both you and your baby is to increase blood volume, both to facilitate circulation of oxygen and nutrients and to help prevent you from going into shock in case of hemorrhage during the birth. Sometimes blood backs up in the extremities, particularly in the legs, and this is how ankle edema results. Nearly 40% of pregnant women experience some swelling at the end of pregnancy; it is a *normal* condition. However, if combined with sudden weight gain, swelling of the face, headache or visual disturbances, report immediately to your care provider.

You can try:

1) Increasing your protein intake.

2) Lying down several time daily, with your feet elevated. It is best to lie on your left side and then elevate your calves and feet with pillows.

3) Changing position frequently during daily activities (avoid standing for long periods).

4) Wearing loose clothing on the legs (no knee-highs or tight nylons).

Avoid:

1) Diuretics of *any* kind, whether medicinal or herbal. Remember that edema is a normal condition. Diuretics will destroy the sodium/potassium balance in your body, and this is dangerous for you and the baby.

SHORTNESS OF BREATH is partly caused by progesterone, which acts on the respiratory center to increase oxygen intake while lowering levels of carbon dioxide (poisonous waste) in the body. In order to accomplish the latter, respirations may speed up and hyperventilation may occur. But the primary cause of shortness of breath at the end of pregnancy is the baby, impinging on the diaphragm and forcing you to breathe more rapidly in order to get enough air.

You can try:

1) Maintaining good posture.

2) Consciously slowing and deepening the breath at the first sign of hyperventilation (begin with a full exhalation).

3) Standing up when feeling breathless and stretching, arms high above your head.

BACKACHE is caused primarily by the growing fetus affecting posture and carriage. Progesterone plays a part in softening the ligaments supporting the uterus so they are more susceptible to overstretching, which causes strain in the adjacent muscles. Unless you pay close attention to maintaining good posture, the weight of the baby will cause sway-back, discomfort and pain.

The problem is intensified if abdominal muscles are lax, because then the uterus will fall farther forward. Excessive bending or lifting heavy objects can also have detrimental effects.

You can try:

1) Using your stomach muscles to hold your posture (you will not hurt the baby by pulling your stomach in).

2) Using appropriate techniques for bending and lifting; i.e., stooping down rather than leaning over, and lifting from this position with your feet far enough apart to give you a solid base of support.

3) Pelvic rocks. These are done by alternately arching the back and straightening it out, and can be performed on hands-and-knees, in a standing position, sitting down (while driving, for example) or lying down on your side. These *really help,* but you must do many repetitions (25-30) to get relief.

4) Wearing low-heeled shoes; high heels accentuate swayback.

5) Adequate pillow support when you rest or sleep.

Avoid:

1) Pain medications of any kind.

LEG CRAMPS are partly due to circulatory disturbances in the legs or pelvis. But since they occur almost exclusively in the last trimester, they are mostly a result of pressure from the enlarged uterus on the nerves running through the pelvic area.

You can try:

1) A change of position.

2) Straightening affected leg, and flexing the foot by pulling toes towards you.

3) Standing on a cold, hard surface.

4) Increasing your calcium intake. For best results calcium should be combined with magnesium; get supplements with a one to two ratio. Vitamin C aids absorption, so take with C tablets or citrus.

5) Increasing potassium intake (good food sources include grapefruit, oranges and bananas).

6) Exercising regularly to promote circulation.

7) Elevating legs periodically throughout the day.

Seldom does a woman experience all of these problems, but a fair number experience more than a few. If symptoms persist, major changes in diet and lifestyle or some emotional reorientation may be required. Time and again, I am moved by the courage of pregnant women; even though birth is a natural event, the adjustment and realignment required in pregnancy are rarely easy. In our culture especially, pregnant women are just not honored and respected as they should be for the task of bringing forth new life.

As labor approaches, many women notice changes that are in fact signals that the baby is about to be born. Emotions run the gamut again, as in early pregnancy. You may feel like being secluded one minute then out and about in a whirlwind of activity the next; like crying one second then suddenly elated for no apparent reason. Needless to say, the hormones have a heyday just before the birth. I've often noticed that when a woman is finally ready, her face has a strained and overburdened look as if overly full of life. Then as labor actually begins, this gives way to a clearer, brighter countenance, partly due to the fact that hormones trigger a last minute loss of up to five pounds of water weight. No one knows exactly why, but many women experience a burst of energy at this time that is almost ecstatic; a feeling of being on top of the world, excited and free. This shifts to a more settled and serious attitude as labor becomes hard work and requires full concentration. It is the hormone *oxytocin* which is responsible for the uterine contractions of labor. Again, no one knows exactly what physiological changes trigger the onset of labor, but we do know that it is oxytocin that keeps it going.

Even though oxytocin is a powerful hormone, it can be affected and even negated by another equally as powerful, *adrenalin*. This is why fear or tension in labor can cause progress to slow or stop. It is not unusual for well-established labor to cease temporarily when a woman arrives at the hospital, or if strangers enter the room and are insensitive or annoying. Of course it all depends on how far along in labor the woman is and how strong her contractions are, but generally, the hormonal actions that maintain labor are more delicately balanced than we think.

On a more technical level, oxytocin causes circulatory changes so that bloodflow is directed to the uterus. Conversely, adrenalin causes a rush of blood to the extremities. Fear initiates this "fight or flight" syndrome, as the body prepares either to do battle or escape from the perception of danger. Stress also causes a release of adrenalin; although levels are lower, the effect is the same overall. If fear in labor becomes extreme, bloodflow to the baby can be affected so greatly that its oxygen levels decrease and fetal distress results. Never underestimate the need for peace and quiet during labor! Try to choose a birthing environment where you will have as few interruptions as possible. A darkened room with just your partner is often ideal.

The discomforts experienced during the birth process are so varied, and so dependent on the specifics of the baby's position, mother's comfort, her environment etc., that discussion of these exceeds the intent of this book. However, in Chapter Nine I will present some birth stories to illustrate the range of sensate possibility in labor. Comfort measures depend on the situation, and although there are some things the mother can do for herself at this point, her main job is to let go and relax and let others minister to her needs.

Many women do not realize that after the birth the most intense physical changes of all will occur, and in a remarkably short time! The uterus shrinks *to the size of a grapefruit* almost immediately after giving birth, and is back to normal in just ten days! The breasts begin to lactate. The body loses excess water retained in pregnancy and the cardiovascular system shifts back to its pre-pregnant state, all quite abruptly. It's no wonder that the new mother needs lots of sleep for the first few weeks!

Let's take a closer look at the hormonal changes postpartum. The moment the baby is born oxytocin rapidly diminishes, although breastfeeding tends to maintain optimal levels during the first few weeks postpartum. And how is this? Nipple stimulation causes oxytocin to release and not only contract the uterus (for firming and toning) but the upper vaginal area as well. This accounts for reports by some women that breastfeeding is an orgasmic experience. Be that as it may, there is no doubt that recuperation for breastfeeding mothers is more rapid than for those who bottle feed. Blood loss is less, and mobility regained sooner.

It is important to understand how overactivity and upset in the first few weeks postpartum can negate these benefits. Just as in labor, any release of adrenalin will inhibit the action of oxytocin. Hence the customs in other cultures (discussed in Chapter One) that place the mother at bedrest for several weeks, or at least offer full support with all physical needs completely covered.

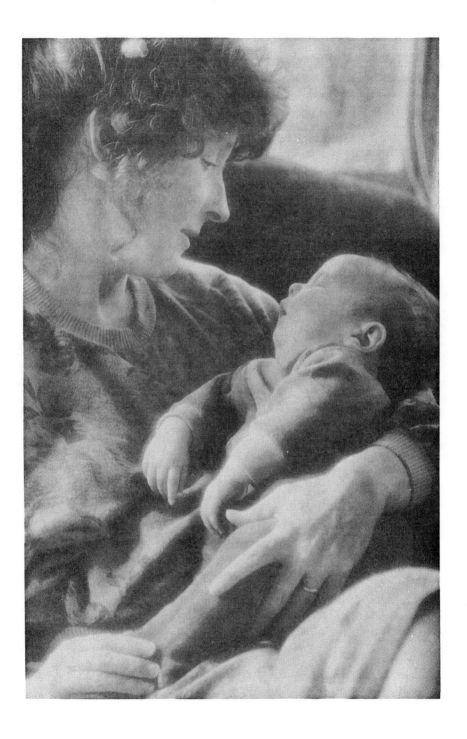

And breastfeeding itself, how is it initiated and maintained? Yet another hormone, called *prolactin*, is responsible. It is thought that high levels of estrogen and progesterone during pregnancy prevent prolactin's release, but when these drop off suddenly with delivery prolactin levels are free to rise. Once breastfeeding is underway, its continuation depends on the sucking stimulus provided by the baby. What this means is that as long as you eat well, rest and take adequate fluids, you will have plenty of milk for as long as the baby nurses, be it six weeks or three years! And the more often the baby nurses, the more milk you will produce. If you have heard stories from friends or family about someone not "having enough milk," she either did not nurse her baby enough, was undernourished or too frightened and nervous to let her milk down.

Yes, it seems that tension not only has an effect on milk production, but on milk secretion. And once more, it is oxytocin that is responsible for triggering the "let down" reflex which starts the milk flowing. This is why a woman having trouble with letting-down may be counseled to nurse alone in a quiet place, or to read something to distract her from worrying, or to have a beer to help her relax.

It is a fascinating point of fact that oxytocin can be released by emotion, by feelings. For example, a woman very excited by her lover may have an orgasm the moment he enters her, with very little physical stimulation. Likewise, a mother can have letdown just thinking about her baby, or upon hearing another baby cry (particularly if hers is not with her at the moment).

If you feel a bit crazy around the time your milk is coming in, don't be alarmed; your hormones are going wild and crying at this point is commonplace. It is often said that letting tears flow helps the milk do likewise. Let yourself go.

Besides these immediate changes, other body systems return to normal within three to six weeks. Stretched and dilated blood vessels regain their tone so that varicosities diminish and swelling is gone. The only persistent reminder of pregnancy may be hemorrhoids, due to localized stress with delivery.

Constipation may also be a problem again, due to a lack of bulk-forming foods or to fear of tearing through stitches if the perineum has been repaired. To return to our earlier format, *you can try:*

1) All of the measures mentioned earlier in the chapter.

2) Pressing a pad of folded tissue against your stitches as you bear down (counterpressure).

Be reassured that stitching is usually several layers deep, and the thread is made to withstand tremendous pressure. The counterpressure you provide is mainly to help you feel more secure so that you can relax.

In general, the postpartum period is a volatile time emotionally. This is due not only to sweeping physiological changes, but also to the psychological impact of becoming a mother and having to accept an utterly new life situation. Even for women with other children, family dynamics are rearranged. This is why honoring basic physical needs is so critical to recuperation; at least if your body is rested and well cared for, you have some stability from which to make the more complex adjustments.

Are you beginning to see how closely the physical and psychological aspects of pregnancy are intertwined? In the next chapter, we'll look at how a woman's response to childbearing is largely dependent on her personality type.

Chapter 4

How We Respond:
Three Typical Patterns

Although we women are complex and unique creatures, with no two of us exactly alike, the basic components are the same for everyone. Physical, emotional and mental qualities blend in a distinctive fashion to make us what we are. And our reactions to the challenges of childbearing largely depend on which of these qualities is strongest in our personality.

Consider the case of one of my former clients, a black belt in karate. Around the beginning of her third month, she became very depressed by the softening of her body, the loosening of her joints. Her emotional expression became strained, stilted. Finally around her 16th week she broke down crying, "My body just doesn't *work* anymore!"

Another client reveled in the heightened sensitivity of pregnancy. Every nuance of feeling was noted, and communicated at length during her checkups. She was so engrossed with her emotions that she often forgot to eat, until finally fatigue and physical complications caught up with her.

Yet another client came to me early in pregnancy already having read nearly a dozen books on the subject! She ate well, went to early pregnancy classes and exercised as directed. However, when asked about her feelings she was always "fine," always in control. Eventually her husband came with her and happened to make a few insensitive comments, at which she suddenly released a torrent of anger and frustration, then broke down and cried.

Each of these women reacted to the challenges of being pregnant very differently. For the first, the fatigue of early pregnancy was the height of frustration, for the second, a good excuse to avoid exercise and for the third, a challenge to her self-control. These three individuals are perfect examples of physical, emotional and mental types.

Let's take a closer, in-depth look at each of these. The PHYSICALLY ORIENTED WOMAN has a vital and animated demeanor. Physical types love to feel in command of their bodies, to use physical expression to push the limits of their thoughts and feelings. They are sensual, enjoying food, drink and other pleasures. They are *initiators;* they love starting new activities but may have trouble sustaining or bringing them to completion.[1] Just because they are physical doesn't necessarily mean they are loose in their bodies, in fact, many use muscle tone and kinetic control as armor to shield them from unwanted emotions or vulnerability.

EMOTIONALLY ORIENTED WOMEN are sensitive, passionate and emotionally self-indulgent. They enjoy exploring the range of their feelings and the effect these have on others. In this respect they may play the role of "drama queen," often prone to exaggeration. Generally quite talkative, they seek an audience for self-validation. They are *sustainers,* so in love with process that they may draw things out unnecessarily[2]. Thus they are not particularly good at bringing to completion or making a fresh start.

The MENTAL TYPE OF WOMAN has a penchant for order. Well organized, well informed and always on top of things, she gives the impression of having it all together when in fact she is simply repressing her feelings and/or desires. Sometimes women of this temperament are overweight, but in this case eating is not a sensual indulgence as much as a way of dealing with frustration. Feelings are just too impossible to organize! As you might suspect, this type of woman is terrific at wrapping things up, tying loose ends together.[3] But knowing full well the magnitude of a looming project, she may have trouble starting up. She may also be frustrated during the course of an activity because she is so meticulous, a perfectionist through and through.

Do you see yourself in any of these examples? Have a hunch now about your basic type? Perhaps you are not as extreme as the above descriptions, since pure types are somewhat rare. Still, most of us have one aspect dominant, the second complimentary to it and the third a bit neglected or undeveloped. In case you are still in doubt (or to make absolutely sure) take the following quiz and see what turns up. Do be honest with your answers; it's pretty easy to fudge this test but you'll get more out of it if you stick to the truth.

PERSONALITY PROFILE

Choose one answer and place a checkmark on the line to the right. Be sure to choose the response that *best represents the way you usually are* (not how you wish you were or think you should be!)

1. *Good organization:*
   a) should arise spontaneously out
      of what I'm doing   ____
   b) is not as important as following
      my feelings   ____
   c) is essential for getting things
      done   ____

2. *I Exercise:*
   a) to keep my body in shape   ____
   b) to get in touch with my feel-
       ings   ____
   c) to maintain good health   ____

3. *My emotions:*
   a) are difficult to manage   ____
   b) are an important part of my life   ____
   c) tend to get in my way   ____

4. *Whenever I feel like crying, I:*
   a) get out and get moving   ____
   b) put on some music and get
       into it   ____
   c) try to control or stop the
       thoughts/feelings that are
       causing it   ____

5. *I generally eat:*
   a) for the way food makes me feel   ____
   b) for the physical effect   ____
   c) to keep myself operative   ____

6. *Doing something new:*
   a) excites me   ____
   b) might be OK if I can get
      around to it   ____
   c) requires some thought for the
      time and energy involved   ____

7. *I prefer to read books:*
   a) short and to the point   ____
   b) that keep me abreast of current
      attitudes and information   ____
   c) if they move or inspire me   ____

8. *Sitting around the house doing nothing:*
   a) disturbs me   ____
   b) is OK once in a while   ____
   c) is something I enjoy   ____

9. *When working on a problem:*
   a) I try to get through it as
      quickly as possible   ____
   b) I find myself going over and
      over it, looking for the key or
      hidden meaning   ____
   c) I organize the facts and seek a
      solution   ____

10. *When it comes to child-rearing, I'll probably:*
    a) look to my highest ideals   ____
    b) see what develops   ____
    c) enjoy teaching my child   ____

11. *When I'm upset, I:*
    a) need to talk about it with
       someone   ____
    b) try to get on to something else ____
    c) expect that feeling will pass
       over, and get back to business   ____

12. *I exaggerate:*
    a) occasionally   ____
    b) more than anyone would
       suspect   ____
    c) almost never   ____

13. *Sentimentality:*
    a) is woven into all I do   ____
    b) slows me down   ____
    c) has little place in my life   ____

14. *Do I need help from others?*
    a) not really, I can take care of myself ____
    b) depends on whether they have anything substantial to offer ____
    c) not unless they truly get involved ____

15. *Whenever I'm sick, I:*
    a) want to withdraw and be left alone ____
    b) try to tough it out, just keep going ____
    c) want someone to talk to and take care of me ____

16. *Strong sensation:*
    a) excites me ____
    b) you mean how I feel? ____
    c) let me think about it . . . ____

17. *A schedule should serve:*
    a) to keep you from forgetting things ____
    b) to charge up your day ____
    c) to help you get things done ____

18. *Other people's feelings:*
    a) are very important to me ____
    b) don't concern me all that much ____
    c) are often unknown to me ____

19. *At a party, I usually:*
    a) go up to people I feel chemis-
       try with ____
    b) emanate feelings to attract
       others to me ____
    c) talk within my pre-established
       circle ____

20. *Most of the time, I drive:*
    a) carefully, efficiently ____
    b) automatically, thinking of other
       things ____
    c) fast but adroitly ____

21. *At a restaurant, I often find:*
    a) that my entree suits me fine ____
    b) that I've ordered too much ____
    c) that I really wanted to order
       something else and now I wish
       I had ____

22. *Skydiving and hangliding:*
    a) would be fun to try sometime ____
    b) are for other people, not me ____
    c) are dangerous and rather fool-
       ish pursuits ____

23. *Completing a project:*
    a) is easy if you just go on to
       something new ____
    b) is difficult, especially if it has
       been enjoyable ____
    c) is challenging, making sure
       everything is wrapped up ____

24. *Structure:*
    a) causes me to rebel   ____
    b) generally escapes me   ____
    c) is my foundation   ____

25. *I think others see me as:*
    a) dynamic, exciting   ____
    b) sensitive, aware   ____
    c) well-organized, "together"   ____

                    TOTALS __ __ __

To score, add up the total checks in each column. If you have the highest number in the left-hand column, your basic orientation to life is physical; if in the center column, emotional; if in the right-hand column, mental.

————————————

Now that you have this information about yourself, what can you do with it? Knowing your basic type will clue you as to how you'll be likely to respond to the transformations of pregnancy and the challenges of birth and parenting. With this, you can tailor your preparation to meet your liabilities head-on, rather than conveniently glossing over them or getting lost in an overly general approach.

A word here about systems in general. This physical-emotional-mental view is just one way of differentiating human behavior. Jung had four types; another system has three categories according to body type. Astrology has twelve signs, and Chinese medicine five elements. None of these need be exclusive of the others, they overlap and combine. *With any system, the most important thing to remember is to use the information not to isolate, separate or limit yourself, but to discover your uniqueness.*

To be perfectly honest, I've always had trouble with systems because they tend to oversimplify what is really complex. On the other hand, this is why they are useful; they break things down and allow certain information to stand out and be clarified. Nevertheless, the temptation to focus only on what is highlighted is very strong. To avoid this, *read all the sections in this book and let the information speak to each part of you.* Discover the fabric of who you are; what is smooth, what is rough and unfinished. Use the information not to reduce, but to add unto yourself!

Now let's take a closer look at each type, in more detail. Please feel free to make notes/personal references in the margins—let this be a workbook for you!

Type One: Physical

As discussed earlier, this woman usually reacts to the changes of early pregnancy with some dismay. Weight gain is disconcerting, but even more so the loss of muscle tone as the body softens in response to hormones. Overall it is loss of physical command that is most disturbing, particularly if this has begun to interfere with the woman's favorite sport or activity. For suggestions on how to manage this, see Chapter Five.

Another complaint from the physical type is the unpredictability of her emotional life. Crying is often viewed as a sign of weakness, a further loss of control. Mostly it's the confusion of strong emotions *interfering with activity,* slowing her down or preventing her from reaching the "highs" or peaks of energy to which she is accustomed (and possibly addicted). Physical types are intensity buffs! The fuzzy, non-focused quality of this phase further adds to their confusion.

Food may also be an issue, as a diet restricted to healthful basics, in large and continual amounts, may seem more a burden than a pleasure. Binging on stimulating foods such as chocolate or sugary pastries is common, in the quest for a rush of energy (again see Chapter Five).

But as pregnancy progresses and the body stabilizes, the physical type may experience a boon of integration, with a new-found emotional dimension. Particularly if her mate is supportive, this can be a marvelous time of ease and richness, an overall loosening up.

As the third trimester approaches, there are new challenges on the physical level. Various discomforts occur as the baby becomes large and heavy, and freedom of movement is restricted. This is a critical phase for the physical type, a time to let her hair down and let others in on her feelings, her needs. This is also the time to discuss expectations and fears regarding the birth itself. Frequently this type plans to "tough it out" in labor and thus may not have developed a birth plan that involves the participation of her attendants. In order to do so she must obtain adequate information and *acknowledge her need for support.* The latter is undoubtedly most difficult for this type but no matter how strong or independent she may ordinarily be, once in labor she must be able to lean on others and let herself be cared for.

Labor will definitely run more smoothly if these adjustments are made in the last trimester, rather than attempted during labor itself. It is much easier to ask for help when you're on top of things than when you are vulnerable and really in need. Practicing while still pregnant makes much more sense than saving all the work for the main event.

If you are the physical type, how do you think you might respond to the first-stage need for letting go? Yes, it can be quite a struggle, since a continual state of passive surrender is hardly your cup of tea! This is not to say that a woman can't be active during first stage; walking, squatting, changing position. But there is no getting around the fact that cervical dilation requires a sustained effort at doing nothing, relaxing fully and completely. If you are impatient and have difficulty following through in general, it's easy to see how first stage might proceed in fits and starts, with alternating periods of rapid dilation and temporary arrest.

What can you do to get yourself through this phase of labor? Here are some hints:

1) *Tell the truth about what you are feeling!* Verbalize discomforts, needs for support or assistance and any ideas about what might help you progress.

2) *Let your hair down completely!* Just because you must relax in labor doesn't mean you can't make noise, or experiment with postures and rhythmic movements.

3) *Let your helpers help you!* Be receptive to their suggestions and assessments. This will be easier if you view the birth as a team effort.

Transition poses challenges for any woman, but for the physical type pressure sensations may be so stimulating that premature pushing results. No way around it; you'll have to *hang loose* until the time is right and the urge completely takes you.

As you might guess, second stage is usually a piece of cake. Physical women *love* to push! They focus the energy of each contraction beautifully, and give it full gusto. Still, the crowning can be difficult; in order to avoid tearing you must *hold back*, although everything inside you is straining to forge ahead.

Once the baby has arrived, postpartum challenges you to respect your need for rest, to accept help from others and to surrender to a fairly monotonous routine of nursing-and-resting, nursing-and-resting for several weeks. This is perhaps the most difficult phase of all. The physical type is definitely prone to overwork, exhaustion and depression. Because of this she is also at risk for infection (due to being rundown).

To keep things on the bright side, she needs enough stimulation to keep her entertained even though she's in bed most of the time. Movies on the VCR, phone chats or brief visits from friends can be tonic. Favorite food treats help too (but watch the chocolate; the baby may react). Nothing is better for relieving tension than a good massage, even if only neck and shoulders. And remember the importance of warmth; keep your feet cozy in socks, the room well heated, etc.

Don't neglect to *line up your support people in advance* to provide these things to you after the birth. And remember that your body will recover better, regain its strength and muscle tone sooner if you do nothing but be with your baby for the first ten days, then gradually resume your normal activities.

Certain exercises can be started just days after the birth, Kegels immediately. Invest in a good childbirth exercise book that includes a section on postpartum work. Before long, your energy level will be up again (although interrupted sleep will affect you for some time to come). For suggestions on newborn care, see Chapter Nine.

Type Two: Emotional

If you're the emotional type, you've probably picked up some clues already on how you might react to pregnancy and birth. The first trimester, with its veritable overload on the feeling level, allows you a heyday as never before. All your emotions are heightened, intensified. Nuances never before experienced may thrill or even frighten you a little. Although this may seem fascinating, your significant others are probably going crazy with your mood swings and you may need to tone it down a bit, particularly if emotional preoccupation is overshadowing physical care. Shake some sense into yourself and focus on your needs for exercise, proper nutrition and adequate rest. Meditation (or quiet time spent collecting yourself) isn't a bad idea either, as this can help you integrate your feeling aspect with the rest of your personality.

In order to decide on an exercise program or nutritional plan, you'll have to collect some information. Emotional types often avoid reading, or else feel that what they do read is either incomplete or inappropriate for them. This is because they tend to hold extreme (or even fanatical) views based solely on their feelings. The critical task for this type is to *actively seek information from a variety of sources, so that fully informed decisions can be made on a somewhat rational basis.*

If this process is begun early in pregnancy, the second trimester can be an absolute pleasure. More than any other type, the emotional woman can *truly enjoy* being pregnant, largely because she finally feels at home in her hormone-intensified state. But enjoyment will be fleeting unless she takes care of her body and makes some concrete plans for the birth and post-partum period.

Assuming she does so, the third trimester poses yet another formidable challenge: letting go of the pregnancy in order to give birth! Yes, the emotional type is loathe to give it up; remember, she's a master at *sustaining* situations! This is why labor often takes a while to get going and why first stage itself may be prolonged, particularly the latent phase when the emotional component has such a strong effect on ebb and flow. What's more, early labor brings an intriguing new level of sensitivity which may cause this type to stall, both to savor her experience and to avoid moving ahead to hard physical work. This is especially likely if she is receiving lots of attention, i.e., people are fussing over her. If this is the case, I generally leave the woman alone with her mate and suggest to family and friends that they step out for a break (get rid of the audience). Sometimes time limits or ultimatums must be given if the woman has been too long without food and/or sleep and is getting exhausted. It's funny, but ultimatums actually appeal to this type as they intensify the drama of the situation!

Once this type settles into first stage she usually dilates beautifully, although emotional conflicts may cause minor arrests from time to time. On the other hand, transition is often rough because the urges to push bring the relative equilibrium of first stage to an abrupt end. Even though first stage is essentially passive it still requires this type to exert more energy than she probably ever has before in her life. And when the pushing urges begin, she may feel forced beyond her capacity. As a matter of fact, emotional women are not overfond of pushing simply because it is so intensely physical. They usually need a lot of guidance to get going and plenty of encouragement to keep at it.

If you are the emotional type, here is a list of things you can do to help your labor run smoothly:

1) Focus on your *sensation*, and play the edges of it by taking on more and more.

2) If you feel yourself being sidetracked by some feeling, *get it out* by telling your mate or helpers. Then focus on your body once again.

3) *Don't be afraid of pushing!* Even though it feels like more than you can possibly handle, just surrender like you did in first stage and your body will do what it should automatically. Only this time, focus your attention downward, through your pelvis and out, rather than trying to rise above your sensation.

4) Don't lose yourself in the feelings and reactions of your helpers. Stick to the business of giving birth.

Postpartum poses challenges similar to those of early pregnancy, especially in terms of physical self-care. Nutrition is more important than ever; a nursing mother needs one-third more calories than she did while pregnant and will be in serious trouble if she neglects to eat. Generally though, the emotional woman has an easy postpartum adjustment in that she tends to rest and breastfeed without much anxiety, as long as she is not getting disturbing messages from friends or relatives. If you are this type, do take care to guard against negative input during the early weeks. You will be *very* impressionable and vulnerable. When in doubt, speak to your birth attendants and seek out the facts.

The same goes with processing any problems or disappointments having to do with the birth itself. Don't give yourself grief by delving into feelings of failure or bitterness; to do so might seriously jeopardize your recuperation. Remember that emotional instability is extreme at this time, and postpone your final analysis for awhile.

For tips on relating to the baby, see Chapter Nine.

Type Three: Mental

This woman is an organizer, an executor; she has very few loose ends in her life and is responsible as can be! Dependable and solid in her sense of self, she is usually quite capable in her worldly role. This is the type who loves to bring things to completion, who enjoys the challenge of fine detail and definitely prefers to be in charge (probably because she's found few people she can trust to do a job as thoroughly as she). Along these lines, she may be somewhat rigid in her manner of operation, her opinions and beliefs. Her emotions are generally kept in check, and her body kept healthy as a matter of course — less from the pleasure of doing so than from the knowledge that it's a good idea.

How do you suppose this type responds to early pregnancy? She may find it disruptive to her usual routine, but as she reads and gathers information she begins to establish new equilibrium. Exercise is undertaken because it is the thing to do, and diet is generally by the book.

The emotions are a little harder to structure! However, if you are this type you've probably learned to view mood-swings as storms to be weathered out. There is obviously some wisdom in this approach, especially in this phase of pregnancy when emotions are so extreme. On the other hand, amidst the turbulence there may be important messages from your sub-conscious that deserve looking into. After all, pregnancy is a time of growth and change. It may be necessary to endure a bit of discomfort and confusion in examining yourself, in order to keep apace with the process.

The challenges of the second trimester are much easier to handle if emotional growth is initiated in the first phase. Once underway, your next task is to *communicate your feelings to others*. This requires that you verbalize emotions, not something you are generally fond of doing but critical preparation for the social aspect of parenting. This may seem unnecessary or embarrass-ing at first, but is essential for finding common ground with other pregnant women. It is *very hard* to parent in isolation; ours is one of the only cultures in the entire world where this occurs!

What happens in the third trimester? Considering that the mental type is good at bringing to completion, it seems reasona-ble to assume that labor would occur right on time. Ah, but the catch is that this type wants to wait until everything is totally ready, and when it comes to making a monumental transition like becoming a parent, the perfect moment may never come! To avoid this, make your nesting preparations as early as pos-sible and set a reasonable limit on additional, last-minute redecorating, refurbishing, etc. You may want to make a list sometime in your sixth or seventh month of all that you con-sider essential, with a separate listing of optional improvements. Then *share* this information with those it may affect, certainly with your partner.

How do you suppose the mental type reacts to early labor once it is underway? Very often she is busy organizing last-minute details, at the same time experimenting with her abil-ity to control herself during contractions. This may lead to a rather long prodromal phase, but as she discovers ways to cope she should make a fairly smooth transition to active labor. In fact, she may progress more rapidly than anyone expects! The remarkable thing about this type is that she seldom requests help during labor and may show no sign of moving right along. I remember attending a birth that was classic in this respect; although my assistant and I were ready and willing to help and her husband was right at her side, the woman refused to be touched, coached or verbally encouraged. It was as though she was laboring alone (although later she said that our mere presence was critical to her confidence). Her husband was so relaxed that he was popping sodas and chatting away while she was nearly in transition! Second stage took some getting used to; one could almost see the wheels turning in her mind as she searched for some point of reference to help her accept the new and intensely physical sensations of this phase. And she did need a bit of direction at this time, in order to shift the focus lower in her body. But once accomplished, she carried on quite independently and gave birth with great dignity.

It is important to note that one of the reasons this woman did so well is that she had a relatively easy, unobstructed labor. Had she required assistance, she might have found it nearly impossible to ask. This is why allowing herself to be vulnerable with others is the number one task for this type during pregnancy.

The opposite extreme from the above example occurs when a woman tries to control labor not by adapting to its demands, but by trying to make it fit some preconceived pattern. Then a veritable battle erupts and the experience can turn into a nightmare. These have been my most frustrating cases, where nothing I can do or say makes any difference. The mind is a powerful instrument; once it is made up it is very difficult to change! If you are the mental type, write up your ideal birth scenario and have your partner do the same. Then compare the two and note the differences, allowing these to suggest yet other possibilities of how labor might unfold. If you can come to see that the perfect birth is not so much a matter of *quantifying* factors (i.e., how long a particular stage lasts or how much control you have) but is rather the result of the *quality* of your relationship to the forces of labor, everything will be easier for you. Being flexible does not mean being helpless! An astute business woman considers all possible pitfalls of a proposal before moving ahead with it; likewise, preparing for all possible eventualities in labor makes for poise and strength no matter what happens.

And how goes the postpartum? The need for rest is usually well accepted by this type, once the rationale is clear. Frequently, the hardest part is coping with the baby. What an unpredictable, uncontrollable and seemingly irrational little being! For suggestions, see Chapter Nine.

Your Weakest Aspect

With the knowledge of your basic type and its vulnerabilities comes the challenge of self-improvement. Most of the suggestions given thus far involve using other parts of your personality to balance any negative or extreme traits of your dominant aspect. Sounds simple enough in theory, but in reality may demand some concentrated effort to bring minor parts into serviceable condition! As mentioned earlier, most women have *one aspect decidedly less developed* than the other two. In general, the most problematic traits of your basic type are a direct result of deficiencies in this area.

For example, a strongly emotional type, lost in dreamy idealism about the "perfect birth," probably has a weak mental side and needs desperately to read for solid information. In other words, if this woman strengthens her mental preparation she will automatically balance her emotional extremism. Likewise, the physical type who always keeps her feelings in check needs to achieve some emotional release in order to ask for help during labor, or to avoid explosive outbursts when parenting.

Check back to the type test earlier in the chapter, only this time note the area with the *lowest* score. When it comes to meaningful preparation for birth and parenting, *it is work on this aspect that means the most.*

In case you need convincing (and none of us savors work in an area we'd just as soon forget!) let's look at this premise in more detail, particularly as it relates to pregnancy. Imagine trying to follow *all* the advice and recommendations you receive from friends and your care provider (not to mention books, magazine articles, films, etc). There simply are not enough hours in the day, and the attempt would be exhausting and stressful. It makes much more sense to focus attention where it is really needed! Besides, this is the only way to achieve optimal health, the key to low-risk pregnancy.

In terms of labor, the work done to balance oneself during pregnancy really pays off. Of course there are no guarantees that even the most thoughtful and thorough preparation will insure an easy birth: there is always a slight possibility of complications that are strictly mechanical and cannot be foreseen. But generally, a woman who is physically fit, emotionally at-ease and fully cognizant of the process she is undergoing will have every advantage for a trouble-free delivery.

Along these lines, never underestimate the physical demands of labor; one source estimates the average energy output for a first birth as equivalent to that of a fifty mile hike! As for the emotions, remember how fear or tension can affect the hormones stimulating labor, even causing contractions to stop altogether. And in terms of mental preparation, consider how understanding the phases of labor and normal reactions at various stages will allow you to keep an overview, no matter what happens. In the event of complications, solid information regarding common practices and procedures can keep you from becoming frightened and help you remain in charge.

Finally, your experience as a parent will be richer and more fulfilling if you are able to respond to the three basic aspects of *your baby's* personality without fear or inhibition. We all want our children to have "the best of everything"; think for a moment on what this really means. A baby needs emotional nurturing, sensitivity to its subtle (and not so subtle!) communication. It needs physical contact via tender touch, confident

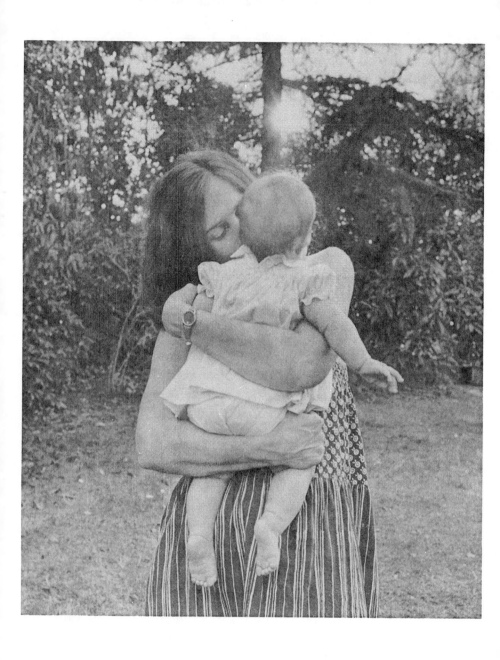

handling, rough-house play and exposure to the great outdoors. And it needs appropriate mental stimulation, with respect to the natural phases of child development. A mighty challenge indeed, but easier and more pleasurable if we are sure of our abilities in each of these critical areas.

One more thing: there are certain benefits in growing to be a more complete and versatile human being that extend beyond the area of childbirth. Even career potential can be positively enhanced by pregnancy, it all depends on how you use it!

In the following chapters on actual preparation, you will find guidelines for physical, emotional and mental types, plus a special "weakest aspect" section. Considering the importance of work in this area, please *read this section first if it applies to you.* Frequently there are long-standing blocks or deep-seated resistance which must be examined before going on to actual practices. In other words, you've got to figure out how your weakest area came to be so in the first place, in order to proceed with meaningful work.

Footnotes:

1. Da Free John, *The Eating Gorilla Comes In Peace: The Transcendental Principle of Life as Applied to Diet and the Regenerating Discipline of True Health.* Dawnhorse Press, San Rafael, 1979.
2. Ibid.
3. Ibid.

Chapter 5

Physical Wellbeing

Conjure up an image of someone in the peak of health. What do you see? Someone fit, energetic, relaxed and physically confident? What are the component parts of this vibrant state of being? On a physical level, at least, they are good nutrition, appropriate exercise and adequate rest.

Actually these three are interdependent; you can't really have one without the others. No exercise program will last long without a diet that provides necessary nutrients; neither can one achieve maximum performance without sufficient rest. Conversely, the best diet in the world may cause excessive weight gain unless enough exercise is taken, and rest is essential to avoid unhealthy food cravings or depletion of reserves. Then again, rest is dependent on release of tension and a healthy nervous system.

Now let's look at the general inclinations of our three basic types with regard to these three components. As you read, concentrate on the material appropriate to your type and as mentioned at the end of the last chapter, read the "weakest aspect" section first if this applies to you.

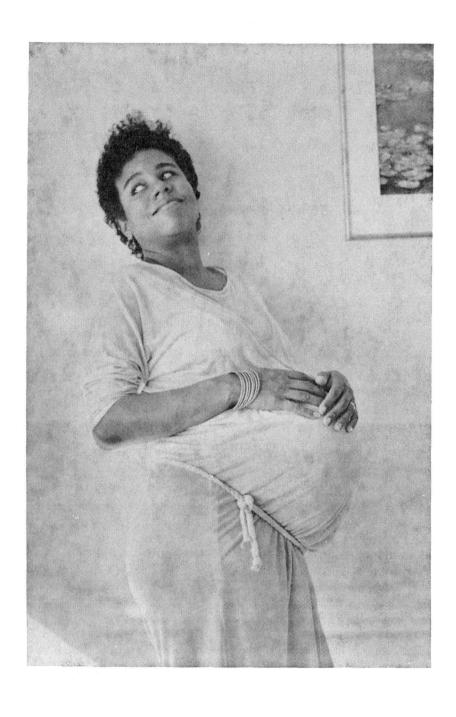

The Physical Type

As discussed in Chapter Four, physical types often enjoy food for its stimulating effect. Routine cravings for chocolate and sugar are typical. If this is you, the easiest way for you to change these habits is to *increase your protein intake,* particularly in the A.M. There is no doubt that caffeine and sugar give you a lift, but this is inevitably followed by severe drop in energy as the effect wears off. If you make the mistake of going back for more of the same, that roller coaster result may disrupt your emotions as well. On the other hand, protein and carbohydrates in healthful, natural foods provide *genuine* energy to your system. These are particularly critical when you are pregnant, as your needs for such are higher to begin with. If you don't get sufficient amounts your body will sound the alarm for fuel, and it is then that the usual indication for empty calories or stimulants must be resisted.

If however you are the athletic type, you've probably learned the importance of good nutrition from sheer necessity and have developed a daily regimen, perhaps involving the use of megavitamins. If so, *be careful* of your dosages of vitamins A and D as these are toxic to the fetus in anything but minimal amounts! Even super high doses of vitamin C can cause withdrawal/scurvy symptoms in the newborn. As you modify your intake it may seem at first that you are losing energy, but as your body adjusts you'll discover renewed vitality. You can avoid withdrawal symptoms by tapering off doses over the span of a week or two.

In general, the physical type must guard against taking good nutrition for granted. Eating "pretty well," or just well enough to maintain the stamina to which you are accustomed, does not necessarily mean you are getting everything the *baby* needs! For example, it is crucial in the first few months when the placenta and fetus are forming to eat *as wide a variety of fruits and vegetables as possible* (or take a multi-vitamin/mineral supplement religiously) in order to meet the complex and ever-changing needs of this developmental phase. And right from the start, you need extra iron and folic acid to make new red cells as your blood volume expands. In the last trimester, your needs for calcium and protein increase dramatically as the baby builds bone and muscle. Iron is even more important at this point since the baby is storing its supply for the first six weeks of life (breast milk has a very low concentration). Invest in a good book on prenatal nutrition and *read it!* Physical types often lack patience with long-winded tomes, so choose one simple and direct.

When it comes to exercise, physical types consider this their greatest strength and herein lies the danger. Particularly in the first trimester, there is a chance that this type will overexert herself and jeopardize the fetus. *Take care that you do not push to the point where your body temperature becomes elevated more than several degrees above normal.* There is evidence that to do so might cause chemical imbalances which could affect your baby's development. A good gauge is your heartrate; even at the peak of aerobic activity it should not exceed 140 beats per minute. If you feel suddenly flushed and thirsty, slow down immediately and have something to drink, or take water frequently during the course of activity as a preventative measure.

However, *do not feel* that you must abruptly change or stop your usual physical routine just because you are pregnant. To do so could seriously disrupt your body's delicate rhythms, and could lead to constipation, stiffness, fatigue or indigestion. Even marathon runners can continue well into pregnancy, although most taper off considerably around the sixth month. By this time the uterus is so enlarged that any impact-causing activity will put excess strain on the supporting ligaments, causing severe shooting pains in the groin or lower back (see illustration III, center insert). Breathlessness may also occur as the uterus begins to impinge on the diaphragm. You may want to consider switching to a prenatal exercise program at this point; sample several until you find one vigorous enough to suit you. Or you might try swimming laps.

Another consideration regarding exercise is what it does (or does not do) to prepare you for labor. Specifically, there are certain muscles that need to be flexible and open, such as those muscles on the inside of the thighs. Pelvic floor, lower back and buttocks should be well-toned but *not tight*, or labor may be obstructed. I have noticed that dancers in particular may have somewhat rigid pelvic tone. You can check for this on yourself by doing perineal massage, as follows:

1) Assume a squatting position, with back support if necessary (you can squat with your back to a wall).

2) Insert your first two fingers into the vagina and contract your muscles around them. Then *release* as fully as possible.

3) See if you are loose enough to insert three fingers. If not, press two fingers down (against pelvic floor muscles) and see if you can find any tight or tense areas. Frequently one side of the musculature is tighter than the other. Wherever you feel tension, massage gently or use steady, increasing pressure until you feel release. Once you've identified tense areas, you may find it easier to massage with your thumb (it's at a better angle than your fingers).

4) Reassess your tension level once again. Contract, then see if you can release to the degree accomplished with massage. If not, work on this every few days, since the ability to release completely is necessary to let the baby descend at birth and to permit the vagina and perineum to stretch without tearing.

To sum up, yoga or deep stretching movements are a necessary complement to any athletic or muscle-building activity.

Remember that the strongest and most responsive muscle is *toned*, not tight!

Deep stretching also lends itself to relaxation and rest. For those of you who are somewhat high-strung, try a stretching routine before bed to help you unwind. Or if restless and wakeful during the night, get up and do yoga before returning to bed.

Another way to get a good night's sleep is to release tension throughout the day so it doesn't build to troublesome levels by evening. Daily exercise is one way to do this, but perhaps your work schedule will not permit it. In this case, try isometric tensing-releasing of major muscle groups periodically throughout the day, with a little deep breathing immediately after to stabilize results.

Emotional release may also be necessary in order to relax. This will be covered in depth in the next chapter; for now, just be aware that it is a significant factor in getting adequate rest.

The Emotional Type

Emotional women frequently have trouble with one or more aspects of physical preparation. Particularly in the early months of pregnancy, this type is usually so engrossed with her personal psychodrama that physical needs are somewhat neglected. Food intake may be either inadequate or so sporadic that she suffers periods of extreme fatigue, exhaustion or even depression.

If this is you, try to think of food as an *ally* for you and the baby. Even if you think you know already, refresh yourself on the four basic food groups and necessary servings of each, then go on to more advanced study. As you research, your greatest challenge will be to remain objective in the face of various approaches until you have read so extensively that you can easily separate the wheat from the chaff, the universal from the salient. *Read, read, read* until you are truly an expert, not just for your own sake but for that of your forthcoming child!

There are several eating disorders that may affect this type. Undereating characterizes the emotional dreamer who enjoys being "out of her body," head in the clouds or immersed in fantasy. For her, adjusting to the heavier and more physical sensations of pregnancy is a tremendous challenge, and eating for two a constant struggle. However, food intake may increase spontaneously if regular exercise is undertaken. Aerobic activity not only stimulates the appetite, it builds strength and endurance needed for labor (and parenting!) Swimming is especially good and often appeals to this type because of the illusion of weightlessness in water.

If this is you, but your schedule will not permit exercise on a regular basis (be honest, now!) you may need to follow a daily diet plan until improved eating habits become routine. This means creating menus for breakfast, lunch, dinner and snacks that will provide your daily requirements. If you are often on the run and seem to forget to eat, carry food with you in your purse or in the car.

If on the other hand you are somewhat overweight and out of shape, you need to examine closely what you eat, and why. If you notice an abundance of "happy food" in your diet, i.e., things that lift your spirits but are not particularly nutritious, you may need to seriously revamp your habits (see the section on sugar, page 63, for suggestions). Again, regular exercise may be the best place to start, although you may need to deal with underlying emotional issues before your efforts will produce lasting results.

Exercise is frequently avoided by the emotional woman, not so much because she is lazy as self-indulgent. More than any other type she is apt to pamper herself while pregnant, and will justify doing so with old-wives' superstitions that any exertion may damage the fetus. But once she gets a taste of *real* exercise, aerobic and stimulating and *fun*, she may quickly grow to love the physical and emotional release, the feeling of self-expression. This type usually loves to dance, and nowadays prenatal dance exercise is available in many locations. Ask your care provider, or call women's clinics for referrals. Then try several programs (if you have a choice) until you find one that appeals to you. Do shop around, because if you don't really like your program you won't stick to it.

And although you may be tempted to quit from time to time (especially towards the end of pregnancy) *don't do it!* Labor will take more stamina than you can imagine, and will take much more out of you if you let yourself get lazy beforehand. Your recuperation will be slower and your postpartum moods more intense. Rest assured that the other women in class sometimes feel like quitting too. Just *take pride* in your body and in what you are doing for your baby!

After the birth, resume exercise gradually. Whatever you do, don't let your body consciousness slip away with the pregnancy; think of what it will take to chase after a two-year old! A fringe benefit of regular exercise is that it is a genuine mood elevator, it keeps you from getting down in the dumps. Put yourself in your child's position and consider this: wouldn't you rather have a Mom who feels bright and happy most of the time than one who is moody or depressed? Besides, if you take care of your own body your child will be likely to follow your example.

When it comes to rest and recuperation, meditation may be your best bet. Emotional women usually need a way to clear out thoughts and feelings in order to really let go. Along these lines, this type often has the mistaken notion that relaxation is simply a matter of lounging about or being lazy, when in fact it takes tremendous discipline to totally still the body. This is particularly true in labor, when fear and anxiety may arise in the face of painful sensation. Meditation prepares you for this, as does self-hypnosis. Investigate both, and try whichever appeals to you.

And practice your progressive relaxation daily! Lie down comfortably, and move gradually through your body releasing feet, calves, knees, thighs, etc. Or try letting everything go at once, a bit more with each exhalation. Sometimes it helps to tense your muscles *before* releasing. These techniques are generally taught in childbirth classes taken during the last few months of pregnancy, but you should begin using them as early as possible if you have a highly emotional nature.

Another marvelous exercise is described by Sheila Kitzinger in her classic book, *The Experience of Childbirth*. She recommends "noticing tension" as it arises in actual life situations. The next time you are under emotional stress (upset, angry, anxious, etc.) notice where you tighten or how you hold your body. Later, when lying down relaxed, recreate the same situation vividly in your mind and see if you can stay relaxed and breathing deeply. This is much like the challenge of labor: learning to meet contractions with welcome and release no matter how frightened or uncomfortable you may feel. Once this letting-go response begins to occur not only during practice sessions but in real life crises, you will have gained a very important skill for coping with the stresses of parenting, relationship and career (not to mention traffic jams, long lines at the bank, etc.).

Actually, this exercise crosses over into emotional preparation. More on this in the next chapter.

The Mental Type

In general, this type has an excellent diet based on solid nutritional information. She usually plans a daily regimen including everything essential, and then sticks to it diligently. This is fine, as far as it goes. But another factor for consideration is the daily fluctuation of nutritional requirements. For example, if the baby is undergoing rapid development and its mother is a bit under the weather, vitamin C requirements, along with B-complex and vitamin E, will probably be higher than usual. All of us have a natural, inner voice of hunger which can tell us what to eat, and when. But this only functions if we are free from addictions to stimulants (like coffee, sugar or caffeine), depressants (like alcohol) or adulterated foods (white flour pastries, chips, etc.). An interesting study was done wherein children given a full range of natural food choices over a period of several weeks were found to eat a well-balanced diet, despite occasional food jags from time to time. For example, one would feast on broccoli exclusively for an entire day, another would eat nothing but apples until dinner. I remember my own kids eating oranges like crazy when they were sick, as many as ten a day!

How to get in touch with this inner voice? Start by asking yourself *before* preparing a meal what you actually feel like eating, and in what amounts. Prepare just that, then while eating check again to see that you take only as much as you *really* want, no more, no less (it's OK to make more if that is what your body signals). Follow this plan for a while and you will definitely experience better health; you may find that you are able to ward off colds and flu before they take hold and that your weight gain will be just right. Being in touch with your body and learning to respect what it is trying to tell you is significant not only for physical wellbeing; we all "hunger" emotionally and mentally too. Learn to recognize the first signs of fear, anxiety, boredom or depression, and use the same attunement to decipher an appropriate response.

Think for a moment on how your inner voice might help you during labor. You can use it to sense which position or breathing to use, when to move about or make sounds, and what to ask of your attendants. In other words, *you will be in control of the situation, even though in a state of physical surrender.* This is the paradox of giving birth, and one of the most important keys to having a positive experience.

Awareness of your inner voice will also make you a better parent. You will be more sensitive to your child's needs, particularly when your little one is in the non-verbal phase and you are feeling (or fumbling) for an appropriate response to crying, restlessness or agitation. I've noticed with my own baby that even as I offer comfort, stimulation, food, etc., part of me watches and fairly well knows already what is wanted. Call this the "higher self" or whatever you will; it can certainly avert stress and struggle and can help foster trust between you and your child.

When it comes to exercise, the mental woman may not be particularly enthusiastic (and that is putting it mildly!). Typically she is a bit uncoordinated, due to her focus "upstairs" and her lack of awareness of gravity. To jump immediately into aerobic activity could result in injury or (heaven forbid) terminal boredom. Before doing anything strenuous or vigorous, this type should explore basic body mechanics: yoga is good for this, as is Tai-Chi. Both teach balance and the interrelation of various muscle groups; they help you find your footing and feel more secure while in motion. You will then be more in touch with the baby, and will probably find greater sensual enjoyment in lovemaking.

Another nice way to get in touch physically is to have massage regularly, at least once a week. Take care to avoid unnecessary talking (although groans, moans or other exclamations are good practice for labor). Giving a massage to your partner can also help you get out of your head.

As your physical confidence grows, more intensive exercise can be undertaken. Using sensitivity as your guide, try whatever appeals to you (swimming, prenatal aerobics, brisk walking, etc.) until you find something to suit. Just take care that your chosen activity is low-impact and at all times modified by any physical discomfort or stress. And make sure you exercise *regularly*; at least three or four times a week for lasting benefit. As the pregnancy progresses, your routine may need modification to adapt to the baby's size or position. The biggest challenge for a mental woman is to *stay flexible and open to change;* not just in terms of exercise but in other areas of her life as well.

Let's return for a moment to the subject of sex. You have probably heard that lovemaking is good preparation for labor, or even that there are similarities between the two. And you may have wondered how something as pleasurable as making love can have anything in common with the reportedly painful experience of giving birth. The connection is that they are both hot, sweaty, intense physical experiences, which can be enhanced by changing position, making noises, releasing your pelvis and inhibitions. If your sex falls a bit short of the above, you might give it a whirl in the name of preparation. You may want to talk to your partner in advance so he can help (or you might simply surprise him!)

Getting control of your vaginal muscles is also important. You will need to release completely to let the baby down and to deliver without tearing. Your muscles must be *well-toned* in order to stretch and give this way.

Begin by doing Kegel's exercise, i.e., contracting and releasing your vaginal muscles. You can do this as you sit on the toilet, stopping and starting the flow of urine. Better yet, put your fingers inside and see if you can contract your muscles around them. This can be done in any position: standing, squatting, lying down. Don't worry if your muscles seem weak or rigid at first, it takes time to develop them. Some women post little "Kegel" signs around the house as reminders to practice. The nice thing is that you can do this exercise anytime, anywhere, and no one will notice. If your muscles are stubborn and inflexible, try a little perineal massage (page 65).

Be sure to resume your Kegels immediately after the birth. And ask your care provider about other postpartum exercises.

Rest and relaxation are critical for the mental type. She is definitely prone to overwork and exhaustion stemming from prolonged concentration. Particularly if she sits at a desk, she may build tremendous tension in her neck, shoulders and lower back. If this is you, a total release and letting-go should be done hourly; it's not even necessary to leave your chair to do this. However, you may find that a standing stretch or a few neck rolls may make your relaxation more pleasurable and refreshing. Just let yourself go completely limp for several minutes, take a few deep breaths and go back to work.

It will probably be necessary to do a more thorough, progressive relaxation in the evening in order to de-brief from the day. Follow the instructions on page 68, but see if you can't

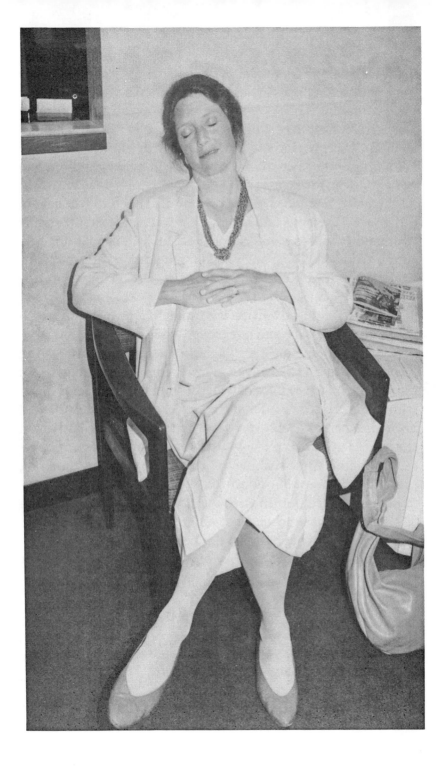

work with a partner, at least in the beginning. The mental type is usually conscientious in her technique but may have some trouble determining if she is truly relaxed. Once you are in position and feel yourself to be fully released, have your partner check by lifting an arm or leg and dropping it (with support). It should fall limply and heavily; if not, you are still holding tension and need to let go even more.

Like the emotional type, you may also need to meditate in order to still thoughts and feelings. Or you may need to *verbalize* your emotions before you can let go. This will benefit not only your physical wellbeing but your communication with your partner and significant others. See Chapter Six for more on this subject.

Mentally-induced tension is a funny thing; you may be feeling pretty good, alert and energized, while actually running on nothing but adrenaline, i.e., "high on stress." It is typical of the mental type to get so involved in intellectual machinations or in carrying out plans by force of will that she completely loses touch with her body. No wonder she may feel disturbed, disoriented or "ineffectual" in a relaxed state! When she lets her guard down she is suddenly vulnerable, so that unwelcome feelings or physical sensations come rushing to her attention. Again, the thing about labor that usually floors this type is that it cannot be controlled, contained or managed; only by surrender to the powers at play can some semblance of order be achieved. The mental type must make it her business during pregnancy to find her personal keys to surrender, be they physical, emotional, mental or all three.

If This Is Your Weakest Aspect

Let's start by considering your upbringing. Were you ever discouraged from physical activity because it might be "dangerous"? Was your family physically reserved, undemonstrative?

Did you or other family members suffer from weight problems? Was sex a taboo subject in your house, an area of repression?

Were you from an intellectual family, who felt that physical activity was unimportant? From a group of sports-nuts, who pushed you so hard you rebelled? Or were you sickly as a child, so that physical activities were automatically curtailed?

If any of these fit your situation, note them on the lines below (your own words are fine).

_____

_____

_____

_____

_____

Now take a moment to write out (briefly) how each of these situations/attitudes from your past has affected you throughout the years. Don't worry about using complete sentences, just jot down your thoughts spontaneously.

_____

_____

_____

_____

_____

_____

_____

_____

_____

_____

_____

_____

_____

Now take these one at a time, and name *one constructive thing* you can do now, in the present, to help yourself get past the problem. Anything that comes to mind is OK (don't second guess your intuition!) If nothing comes to mind yet, don't worry; give it a day or two.

_____

_____

_____

_____

_____

_____

_____

_____

_____

_____

_____

_____

_____

Perhaps you can see already that you have your own resources for handling some of your problems. Or if it seems that making changes is easier said than done, you may need additional help from a counselor or support group (more on this as we go along). But first, let's take a closer look at some of these problem areas in more detail.

If you suffer from serious eating disorders such as anorexia (self-starvation), bulimia (binging and purging) or extreme obesity, you probably have emotional issues that you've not handled or openly confronted. The interesting thing is that you may have *inherited* these emotional issues from your parents, without ever having experienced the situations that caused them to arise in the first place. In other words, the underlying problems are not really *your own*. Think about this for a moment. See if you can identify any highly charged feelings transmitted to you.

If so, you may be able to *disown* these reactionary attitudes that don't really belong to you. Declare your independence now, and in all future interactions with your parents. You may need to see a counselor to help you sort things out or consolidate your decision to be free, but at least you can initiate the process.

There are also fine support groups for women with eating disorders. Even if you have your food intake under control, it is critical that you look at the issues that caused your problem initially or you may inadvertently pass these along to your own child.

There are other less severe eating disorders which nevertheless threaten pregnancy. If you are one who survives on a diet of junk food or mediocre restaurant fare, you may be passing some dangerous additives and preservatives on to your baby. Or if you go for long periods without eating, then binge on less than nutritious foods, you may be depriving your baby of nutrients critical to normal development. In either case you will probably suffer from nausea, indigestion, constipation or heartburn. It is especially critical in early pregnancy that you eat as wide a variety of healthful foods as possible, particularly fruits and vegetables, to supply your baby with the trace nutrients needed for basic development. Supplements help, but they do *not* provide additional calories needed for increased metabolic function. Be sure to read the section in this chapter on natural hunger (page 69). This should help you get a handle on an erratic, jaded or compulsive appetite without unnecessary struggle.

Let's move on to resistance in the area of physical activity/exercise. If this is you, *begin with something you like doing and feel safe with.* Pursue anything for which you have some natural talent or ability, be it dancing, swimming or hiking. Start out slowly and don't push for results, otherwise you will get discouraged and may have to start all over again.

Sometimes women avoid exercise because it causes the release of pent-up emotions. I can remember days in my prenatal aerobics class when after a fight with my husband, I suddenly began crying as the energy reached an intensity where I could once again feel my anger or pain. Could you be avoiding exercise because you have feelings you don't wish to confront? If so, rest assured that vigorous exercise is one of the healthiest and *least destructive* ways to discharge emotion. Not that you won't have remnants to deal with later, but at least you will be in the driver's seat.

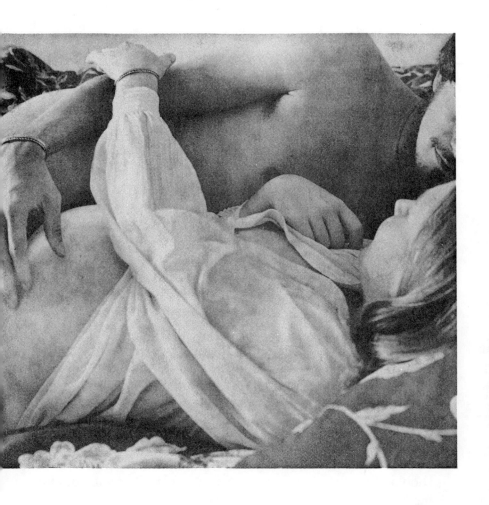

Problems with sex and physical intimacy are often complex and are therefore a bit beyond the scope of this book. Counseling is almost always critical, particularly if there is history of sexual abuse. As a women's healthcare worker, I've learned that scars from abuse run very deep and may take years to heal. The same goes for victims of incest, domestic violence, etc. Start by contacting an organization that deals with your specific problem; they can refer you to a counselor who is an expert in the field.

If sex is something you've never really enjoyed, perhaps you should discuss this in depth with your partner. Ask first if he's willing to help, support or just listen to you; whatever it will take to launch this delicate discussion. Maybe he has hangups too, and you both should see a counselor. Often there's some problem with foreplay; the woman feels she needs more in order to let go, the man feels uncomfortable with the intimacy it creates. But the fact remains that women *need* foreplay to achieve orgasm. Despite the difficulty, it's best to broach the subject now so the sexual intensity at birth doesn't throw you both for a loop.

If your sexuality has been somewhat repressed over a period of time, you probably have some problems with your self-image. Help yourself to a little pleasure; take a sauna, get a massage or otherwise adorn yourself with lotions, treatments, etc. You should also masturbate whenever you feel like it; it will not hurt the baby. Try dressing according to your mood, everything from wild to conservative. And have someone take pictures of you in all your pregnant glory: although you may feel awkward and think yourself unattractive, you'll probably be surprised how good you look and will definitely treasure these in later years.

If you're the type who has problems with chronic tension and stress, take a good long look at yourself in the mirror. What is tension doing to your face, shoulders, hips, posture? See for yourself the importance of finding a better way of being. If you are an overachiever, constantly pushing for excellence, ask yourself *why* you feel compelled to work so hard or struggle so

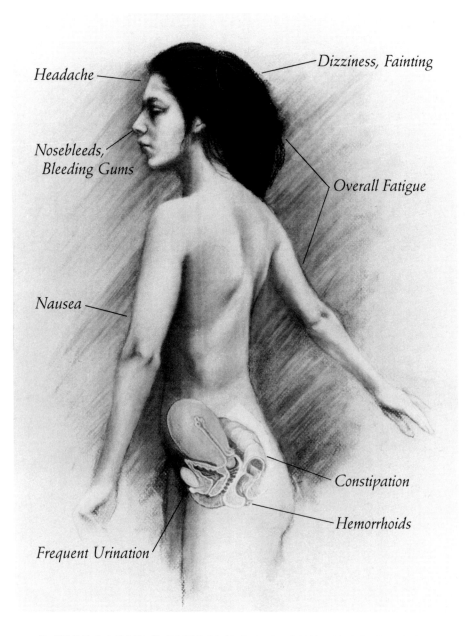

Headache

Dizziness, Fainting

Nosebleeds,
Bleeding Gums

Overall Fatigue

Nausea

Constipation

Hemorrhoids

Frequent Urination

I. HORMONAL EFFECTS IN EARLY PREGNANCY

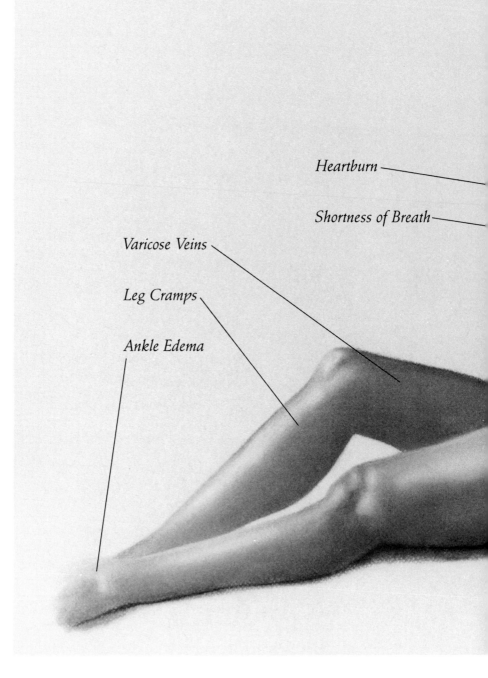

Heartburn ——————

Shortness of Breath ——————

Varicose Veins

Leg Cramps

Ankle Edema

II. PHYSICAL DISCOMFORTS OF LATE PREGNANCY

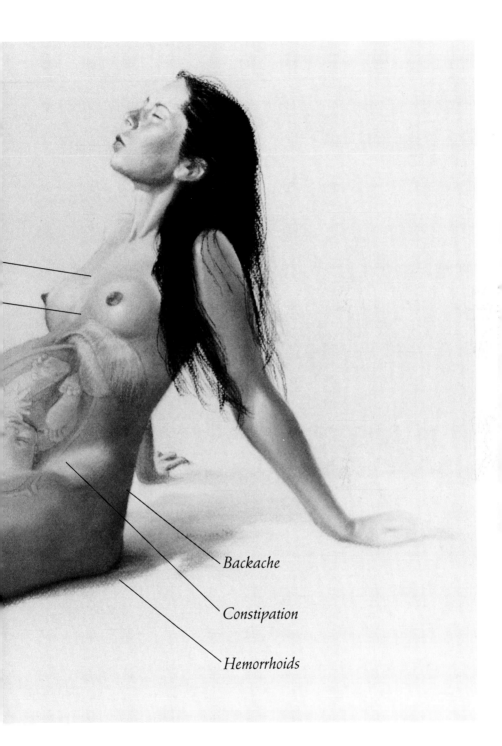

Backache

Constipation

Hemorrhoids

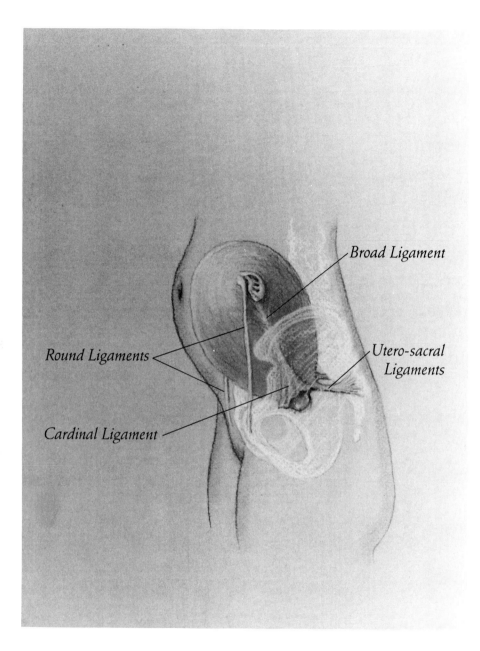

Broad Ligament

Round Ligaments

Utero-sacral Ligaments

Cardinal Ligament

III. LIGAMENT SUPPORT OF PREGNANT UTERUS

continuously. Re-read the first chapter of this book, and reconsider the nature of perfection. In my own experience of nearly forty years, with three children and several successful careers in place, I find the struggle for equilibrium ongoing. I have learned the hard way that you definitely cannot isolate work-related problems from the rest of your life. Eventually these catch up with you, whether by nervous breakdown or debilitating illness. Put another way, the body has its own means of restoring balance, in spite of what we will or desire.

Underlying the overachiever's apparent self-confidence may be a serious sense of inadequacy. Often this type works and slaves just to keep this below the surface. Hypnosis can be of tremendous help, as healing can take place without a lot of conscious struggle. Whatever the method used, it is *very important* to address this problem during pregnancy, since labor will invariably lift the lid on any emotions a woman has been keeping at bay. Last-minute processing may cause progress to slow or stop, or may even lead to Cesarean.

But don't despair; whatever your difficulty, help is out there waiting for you! Everyone has problems; the real test of character is whether you've got the courage and commitment to look for solutions.

One more leading question for the workaholic. How well can you play and have a good time? Make it your business in pregnancy to have fun *at least once a day*. This may not be easy at first; you may really have to make an effort. But after a while it will come naturally. All other therapies aside, laughter may be your best medicine.

Chapter 6

Emotional Health

An emotionally healthy woman is a bit harder to identify than one who is physically fit. It takes awhile to get to know someone well enough to assess their emotional equilibrium, to have a clear sense of what they're all about. How would you characterize an emotionally healthy woman? Self-confident? Strong but flexible? Warm and receptive yet self-contained?

Contrary to what you may believe, the woman with these qualities is neither lucky or born that way. Especially in these times of social upheaval and rapidly fluctuating mores, just about everyone has had to work to preserve their emotional stability. Sometimes this means therapy, sometimes being painfully honest about problems with relationships or one's career. Whatever the means, suffice to say that even the most natural and spontaneous personality has probably had some struggle to get that way.

To understand why this is so, consider how confusing social programming has been for women over the past twenty years. Sexual mores have swung 180 degrees, from free-love to celibate courtship. Woman's role in the workplace still ranges from restricted access to full (or overtime) participation. Most of us now juggle career, parenting, relationship, housekeeping, entertaining, etc. as never before. Even in terms of fashion, we've gone from the mini to midi and back again, from the "natural look" to the most artificial and extreme "punk" styles. Let's face it, we women ride a rollercoaster of fads and fancies dictated largely by men, or at least by a very materialistic culture. Even the most secure little girl goes temporarily crazy during adolescence over her self-image. And after a few experiences of sexual harassment, discrimination in the workplace or disappointing attempts at long-term love, it's no wonder that counseling (or something equivalent) becomes necessary to regain a sense of self-worth.

Apart from the struggles of coming-of-age, there are others which can strain even the most stable personality, particularly while pregnant. Marital difficulties, stress at work, family illness or estrangement are all extremely trying in the best of circumstances, but even more so in the face of hormone changes, physical discomforts and major adjustments in lifestyle.

Marital (or relationship) difficulties deserve special attention if compounded by pregnancy. It is very difficult to share birth with your partner if you both feel alienated, and the postpartum period (which is stressful anyway) is apt to be the last straw. If such is your situation, counseling is an absolute must: as painful as it may be, you deserve to know *before* the baby comes whether to seriously plan for single-parenthood. You would certainly need to develop a more extensive support system, might consider relocating and would need to revamp your finances. By all means, set wishful thinking aside and force the issue; this will be best for everyone in the long run.

Career-related stress should also be handled during pregnancy so that it won't reassert itself later when the added responsibilities of mothering make it even more difficult to cope. If you are generally overburdened, perhaps you might arrange shift-sharing or could press for a more equitable distribution of responsibility. If there are difficulties with your environment or associates, go ahead and confront the situation. Again, it is

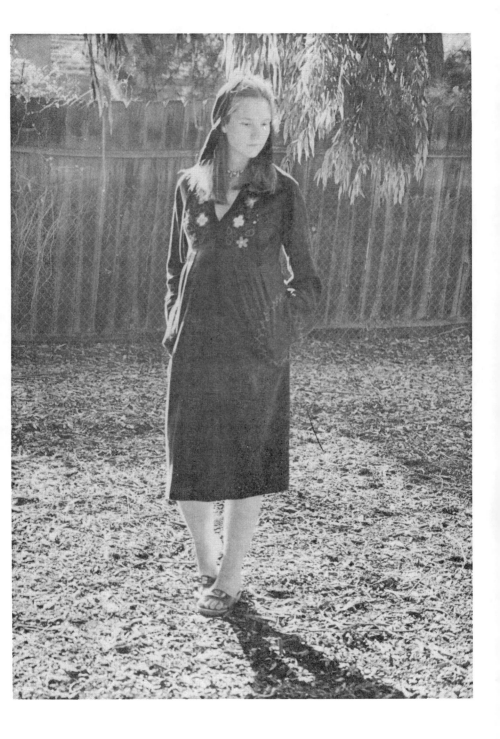

better to find out while pregnant if problems are insurmountable so that you can make alternative plans. But do give it your best shot, and try to be optimistic in the face of conflict. It may take days for the dust to settle after discussion, and weeks for a final agreement to be reached.

If someone in your family is seriously ill or close to death, you must at all costs avoid assuming the burden for other family members. To do so could jeopardize the pregnancy. It has been my experience that the stress of maintaining a day-to-day vigil necessitates a good deal of emotion de-briefing and regular physical release. Massage is especially good because it eases and rejuvenates simultaneously. Above all, protect yourself and your little one from excessive strain.

Always keep in mind when addressing these problems that pregnancy adds its own special effects. As a channel for new life, for creative forces both powerful and tempestuous, you are bound to fall apart now and then, lose your temper or get the blues. There is certainly *nothing wrong* with seeking help when in a state of crisis. Frequently, pregnant women feel immensely frustrated at their vulnerability and lack of control in handling their difficulties; they feel as though they've lost something in becoming pregnant that may never be regained. Actually the reverse is true; there is an overload of energy, a literal and figurative gain that makes for more than can be managed at times. Pregnant women should be honored and respected for taking this burden, but in our culture the opposite is often true. Therefore, do your best to *honor and respect yourself,* especially if the going gets rough.

Now, some specific guidelines for each basic type.

The Physical Type

As mentioned earlier, this type has the tendency to control the emotions. Rather than letting herself be vulnerable to feelings as they arise, she tends to sublimate them in physical activity or rebuff them with physical armor. Either way, her emotions are not as spontaneous or free-flowing as they need to be for giving birth or parenting. This type also uses her feelings to create or intensify sensation, rather than letting them have their own integrity. Consequently she may miss altogether their underlying cause or meaning.

If this sounds like you, try keeping a daily diary of emotions, writing them down as they arise. It's best to have a purse-sized notebook for this purpose, but even if you jot them on scraps of paper at first that's OK; the main thing is to *write them down*. For example, over the course of a day you might feel anger, frustration, jealousy, anger again, sadness, confusion, excitement, happiness, concern, anxiety, etc., etc. After several days have gone by, notice which feelings predominate and think back on the situations which caused these feelings to arise. If your life runs like a broken record, you may need to make some major changes in your routine. Or perhaps you notice that seemingly unrelated events are all causing the same emotional reaction. For example, waiting at the bank, talking to your mother, shopping for shoes and making dinner all make you feel angry. If so, there is probably an underlying cause that you haven't examined. Maybe it all has to do with some situation at work, or a problem in your marriage. If you can just figure out what the *real* issue is, you've got it half-licked. Then you can take charge of your situation rather than being its emotional victim.

If you feel stuck or uncertain, you might want to see a counselor for help. Counseling with a focus is very different than long-term psychotherapy and may require only a few sessions. By all means take a chance and try it, you have nothing to lose and much to gain.

Another major issue for the physical type is accepting support from others. As mentioned in Chapter Three, it is critical to articulate hopes, fears and expectations to those who will attend the birth. Here again is the issue of vulnerability. Although you may be used to doing things your own way, in your own time, labor will force you to rely on those around you. You are going to have to let your body *go*, which may mean leaning on others, feeling dependent or even breaking down completely. This may be hard for you to picture now, but if/when the time comes, wouldn't you rather avoid a scene? If there is anyone you've invited to the birth with whom you have no real intimacy, better reconsider now.

The same goes for your care provider(s). Can you let your hair down with them? If not, do you have enough support otherwise to make up for it? Remember, you have nothing to prove to your provider! You are paying them to assist you, and contrary to what you may envision, the time may come when you feel at the mercy of their assessments or recommendations. If this image does not sit well with you, insist on time at your next checkup to talk. It is never too late to change providers!

When it comes to parenting, you may find it very difficult to be continually patient and giving. You won't be able to run around on your own time anymore, and will need to rely on others to assist you. Think for a moment: who are these people? Has anyone offered to help after the birth? How do you feel about having them in close quarters at a time when you will be extremely vulnerable? Be realistic regarding your emotional limits when it comes to casual acquaintances. But do keep an open mind (and heart) for family members. Giving birth will affect your blood relationships in ways that are difficult to fathom until you've been through it.

Along these lines, perhaps you've been thinking about your mother a lot and find yourself trying to communicate at deeper levels. This is natural, and although it may be painful for you sometimes, keep trying. Your mother can provide a very special kind of support postpartum that is worth working for.

It is said that a child opens your heart to humanity. Let this process begin for you during pregnancy; you'll be on the right track!

The Emotional Type

What does an emotional woman have to learn about being emotional? Plenty! Let's consider first the type who has no trouble expressing her feelings but tends to be insensitive to the needs of those around her. Here's our drama-queen again, apt to run over others with her own intensity. Thus she may turn away her strongest supporters: her partner, best friend, other family members, even her care provider. And without support, both labor and the early months of parenting will be difficult at best. This type needs to learn that emanating an emotion is not the same as discussing it objectively! She must teach herself to still the emotional whirlwind long enough to get at the real issues.

It is a great weakness of this type that she expects others to know what she is feeling, and unless they respond according to her desires she may withdraw in anger and resentment, without the other party having any idea of what is going on. I cannot stress enough the importance of *putting feelings into words*, in terms of preparing for labor and effective co-parenting! Although she may be virtually psychic at times, just as often the emotional woman *projects* her feelings onto others and utterly confuses the situation.

The underlying issue here is power. This type tends to think she will somehow diminish herself by speaking out, that words are just not adequate to express what she feels, but in reality may be hoarding the power of her feelings as a means of controlling the situation.

If this sounds like you, and you find that these tendencies have become habitual, you may have a tough time getting anywhere in conversation. Try focusing on what you think for a change, rather than on your emotional reactions to what others do or say. Then work on *owning* your feelings, i.e., "I feel _____" rather than "You did _____ to me."

This is critical to receiving support during labor. Unless you share your vital self with significant others in a direct and above-board fashion, they will never be able to assist you as you'd like. If you feel stuck in this pattern and don't know where to turn, counseling might be the answer. See if your partner will go along with you. It is worth the initial exposure and discomfort to have a chance at getting what you want in life.

And then there are the emotional types who are *overly* sensitive to the feelings of those around them, who tend to negate their own emotions even though in touch with them. This is the martyr syndrome, which has as its base the same play of hoarding power by holding emotions back. Only this type will turn the power not only against her partner, but against herself as well.

She too needs to work on articulating her feelings, but should focus primarily on *self-containment*. This means learning to separate the threads of her own feelings from those belonging to others. This will be absolutely critical in labor. Picture twelve hours of hard effort, with attendants becoming tired, tense or anxious; if you are swept away by their reactions, your progress may slow or stop altogether. The best way to separate yourself from those around you is to *strengthen yourself from the inside out.* For example, say your husband comes home from work cranky, emitting feelings of inadequacy and anxiety and suddenly *you* find yourself wondering why you can never make him happy or how it is you've lost your ability to charm and thrill him. In short, you've just inherited his problem day, kit and kaboodle! Do the both of you a favor and *just drop it.* Instead, look at what you are feeling inside, at your own state of being. If the feeling is positive, i.e., happy, contented, loving, let it flow from your heart until you feel it emanating. This may automatically put your husband back on track, but that's not the issue. The point is that you needn't be dragged down by those around you. If on the other hand the feeling inside you happens to be negative, *leave the room* or you may very well have a serious argument. Once alone, take a closer look at what's going on and either think it through or let it go, as seems appropriate.

The overly sensitive type may also have problems postpartum. She may be so impressionable and vulnerable to the thoughts and opinions of others as to feel her identity slipping away. If this is you, think carefully about whom you wish to see after the baby is born. Share yourself only to the point where you feel your strength beginning to lag, and then say in a loud, clear voice, "I'm sorry but I am tired and need to be alone now." Practice saying this a few times right now (if you are true to character you may never have said this before!).

You may also need to use the aforementioned self-strengthening technique in caring for your baby. Especially if your little one is crying inconsolably, let not your heart be broken! Just radiate whatever good you can, or have your partner or a friend relieve you as you leave the room to get yourself back together. In fact, this technique may become a permanent part of your parenting bag-of-tricks; it is especially useful when your child reaches adolescence! More on coping with baby in Chapter Nine.

The Mental Type

Mental women often have their greatest difficulty with the emotional aspect. This is because emotions are so unpredictable, unruly and seemingly unproductive. The trick is to see that emotions can enhance the quality of life overall. They can provide information essential for making important decisions. And they can positively affect physical health and wellbeing.

If you have problems expressing your emotions or don't feel particularly in touch with them, you might try following the suggestion given earlier in this chapter for the physical type, i.e., begin noticing your feelings and jotting them down as they arise. Because mental women by nature enjoy making lists, you will probably find this easy to do. But take it a bit further on day two and try to discover the source of your feelings. Write this out using this format: "I am angry because _____ _____" or, "I am elated because_____ _____." This way you can use your analytical abilities to discern the emotional fabric of your day-to-day life.

Although we are accustomed to thinking of emotion as *response,* our feelings may also *cause* situations to develop. For example, say you've been angry with your boss for the past few days and when your husband complains about dinner being late, you argue violently. Here pre-existing feelings caused an event to occur that might otherwise not have happened. It is especially critical that the mental type stay alerted for this configuration; she tends to give so little credence to her feelings that she is unaware of their power, for good or ill.

After several days of charting your emotional life, you will begin to see that you can use your feelings either positively or negatively. You may also choose to surrender to an emotional intensity that frightened you before, once you see the overall pattern and feel secure in its scope. Eventually you may embrace your emotional self fully. To do so would certainly make you a more understanding and responsive parent.

One of the greatest challenges for the mental type is to allow others to participate in the structure of her life. Highly independent and generally impatient with others' less efficient ways of being, she is basically convinced that the only way to get things done is on her own. Unfortunately, this does not hold true for giving birth. Unless you have a textbook labor, you may well require more help than you've ever needed before in your life! Obviously you must prepare for this somehow. For starters, take what you have learned about your emotional nature, particularly how you respond to stress or upset, and consider how each person you've invited to the birth might help you cope. Get specific; perhaps your best friend could rub your shoulders, your husband hold your feet and look into your eyes, your sister come in every now and then with some words to make you smile. Go ahead and plan the event to suit your fancy. If in your contemplation there is someone who doesn't seem to belong, by all means let them know that you've changed your mind. This can be done tactfully and without hurting feelings if you just say, "I've reconsidered having a lot of people at the birth, and would like to wait until I'm in labor before I decide."

Carry this projection of friends' and relatives' participation over to your postpartum phase. Again, ask yourself if there is anyone you'd rather not see at this vulnerable time, then consider specific roles for your chosen helpers.

As mentioned before, baby care may be quite a challenge for you. No matter how well you organize your postpartum support system, that little one will foil every premature attempt at establishing a routine. But if you use your pregnancy to develop emotionally, and carry through during the birth, surrendering to the baby's needs won't be all that difficult.

If This Is Your Weakest Aspect

We humans are by nature highly emotional creatures. If this side of you is repressed, chances are something very disturbing or distressing happened to you in the past. But rather than hunting around for the exact cause, try looking more closely at how you are feeling now, in the present.

If you begin with the exercise on noticing and writing down your feelings (detailed on page 87) you will probably find that your most prevalent emotion is anger. This is natural for one who has been holding feelings in for a long time. So take the bull by the horns, and do some work on your anger directly. Fill in the section below as fully as you can (you can use extra paper if needed).

I am angry at _____

because _____

_____.

I am angry at_____

because _____

_____.

I am angry at_____

because _____

_____.

I am angry at_____

because _____

_____.

I am angry at_____

because _____

_____.

At this point, don't worry if you find yourself going back in time. With a focused way of dealing with your findings, it is appropriate.

The other side of anger is *forgiveness*. This will be of benefit not only to the recipient of your wrath, but to you as well. Forgiveness is the only way to heal the part of yourself that is still hurting. With the following exercise, you may find you want to focus on a particular individual (perhaps one of your parents) and forgive them for the many things they did (or didn't do) throughout the years. If this seems a bit silly to you at first, just think: here's a chance to put into words how you *really feel* and get it out of your system!

I forgive _____

for _____

_____.

I forgive _____

for _____

_____.

I forgive _____

for _____

_____.

I forgive _____

for _____

_____.

I forgive _____

for _____

_____.

If anger has become a habit for you, you may need to do this daily until you discover new ways of coping. Remember that there is *nothing wrong* with getting angry; it's what we do with it that counts! The best way to handle angry feelings is to communicate them directly to the source, before they become explosive or violent. This sounds so easy, but is actually one

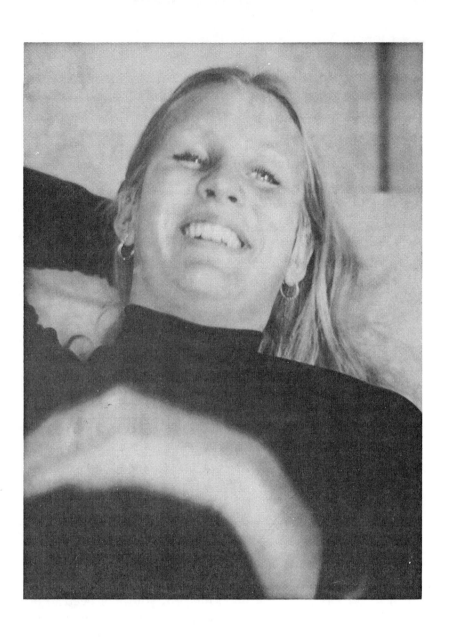

of life's toughest assignments. To tell a loved one you are angry at them makes you very vulnerable, whereas holding back can give you a sense of control, of being in charge. The trouble with this is that the other person has no idea what's bothering you, and so may persist until your anger reaches uncontrollable levels. Stop for a moment, and think what kind of parent this behavior would make you, and I think you'll see the need to start working on this as soon as possible.

Once you admit your anger, you begin to move past it. Then you will be able to feel a wider range of emotions, though not all necessarily pleasant at first. You may experience sadness, loss, anxiety, frustration, desperation, even depression. But at least you may be comforted by the fact that *everyone* has these feelings! Despite what you see in the movies or on television, we all get blue sometimes and are each responsible for figuring out what to do about it.

If in the course of your work on anger you have found something deeply disturbing, i.e., an incident when you were battered or abused, abandoned or victimized, you may need the help of a professional counselor to regain your self-esteem. Ask your care provider for referrals, or look in the phone book for organizations dealing with your specific problem.

From here on in, work can become play. Emotions can begin to enhance the quality of your life, you can reclaim your humanity and enjoy sharing with others the spoken or non-verbal expression of feeling. Think what this will mean for you and your child. You two are going to have a *good time* together!

Chapter 7

Mental Preparation

How do we recognize the woman who is mentally prepared for birth and parenting? She is *well-informed*, i.e., she has actively sought out information specific to her concerns. She is *decisive*, i.e., she knows where she stands on certain issues, what she does and does not want. She is *communicative*, i.e., she informs those most likely to be affected of her plans and preparations. And she is *creative in her thinking*, i.e., she is able to improvise on her knowledge, to expand on what she has learned and adapt to a variety of situations.

Let's consider these abilities one at a time. In terms of becoming well-informed, the obvious sources include books, articles, films and videos. But another critical avenue of learning is dialogue and discussion with others. Being well-informed not only involves reviewing current information, but consulting experts for their seasoned opinions. Particularly if the subject is one with which you have no first-hand knowledge, it is essential to get perspective from someone with experience in that area.

Say, for example, that you are suffering from morning sickness. You have read several books for general advice and have

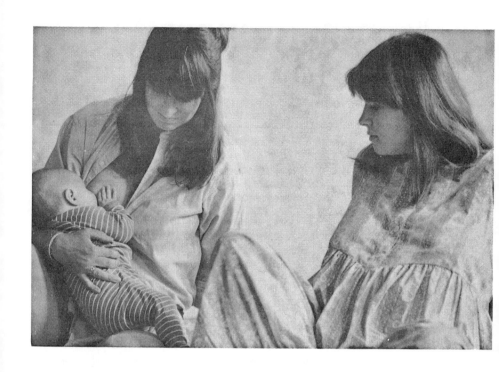

phoned your care provider for suggestions. But you might also call one or two good friends who have recently been pregnant, to find out what they tried and what did and didn't work for them. On the basis of your differences and similarities, getting a sense of what would be most likely to work for you shouldn't be all that difficult.

Another critical component in making appropriate decisions is self-awareness. Unless one has some focus of inquiry and continually checks to see if data is applicable, it is easy to become overwhelmed in the course of gathering information. Granted, there is a fine line here with regard to maintaining an open mind. But there must be some sort-as-you-go process for most of us, or we reach overload before all the facts are in.

It helps to evaluate your source objectively before adopting any information as your own. Get in the habit of reading the author's preface or introductory statement; if his/her basic orientation is at odds with your own philosophy, the information presented may be interesting but not particularly relevant to you. And when consulting a friend or other person for their opinion, consider their biases and be sure they are answering your question specifically, since the tendency to be tangent is strong in all of us. Sometimes an otherwise trusted confidant is simply unable to help; they either lack the experience or would rather not discuss the issue. In this case, take care to disregard unsolicited advice or projection.

The key to being decisive is having adequate information, getting *all* the facts. This may take some time, and more than a little patience. In the meanwhile, it helps to formulate and articulate all you *do* know, so your gains aren't swept away by the tide of oncoming information.

The ability to educate yourself and make decisions won't really amount to much unless you are able to gain consensus with those on whom you must depend. Communication is critical for developing realistic plans, and for keeping those plans up-to-date. Sometimes we make the mistake of thinking that simply by informing others of our needs and desires, everything is settled. But unless we are aware of their response and come to agreement, our plans may fall apart at the crucial moment. This is why it is so important to have open and repeated discussion with one's care provider *in advance* of the birth!

The ability to think creatively ties everything together. Mental flexibility allows us to circumvent obstacles, or to adapt them long enough to discover alternatives. Unfortunately, most of us require study at the school of "hard knocks" or must suffer repeated encounters with Murphy's Law before developing in this respect. Learning to expect the unexpected is merely a start; it's what we *do* with it that makes a difference!

Creative problem-solving requires an ability to go beyond the simple collection of facts to a synthesis all one's own. This is especially critical if you get stuck during labor, or if nothing you have read seems to work in caring for your child. *The key to cultivating creative thought is to set aside fear and stability for a search of the horizon.* It means taking risks, but these can be calculated on the basis of what you know already. It means having faith in yourself, not minding the occasional deadend. It takes surrender to the current of pure thought, and requires an ability to steer a clear course through conflicting information. And it necessitates knowing when to stop and consolidate your learning for re-evaluation.

All of this will seem less abstract if we follow the case of a woman stuggling to develop these abilities during the course of her pregnancy. Let's take the example of Sara, 28 years old and expecting her first baby. She is five months pregnant, and is planning to give birth in the hospital.

Sara is concerned that there be as few interventions as possible, particularly those that might adversely affect the baby. She begins by purchasing several books with specific sections on what to do in case of complications. Although a bit hesitant at first, she talks to new mothers in the store or on the street about their births, trying to understand how these complications arise and what can be done to prevent them. She tries asking her doctor, but there is little time for discussion at prenatal visits.

Sara then speaks to an old friend long-distance, who describes her birth in vivid detail and sings the praises of the alternative birth center where she gave birth. Intrigued and curiously elated, Sara pursues this option, checking first to see if her hospital has an ABC and whether or not her doctor will let her use it. She talks it over with her husband, and together they tour the facilities. While there, Sara is introduced to a midwife doing births at the center, whom she likes very much. Upon inquiring, she discovers that midwives assist nearly 75% of the deliveries there.

Sara continues her research. She learns that interventions are much more likely to occur in standard labor and delivery facilities than in alternative birth centers. Part of the reason, she discovers, is that women qualified to use these facilities must be low-risk to begin with and are therefore less likely to develop complications. But she also learns that good prenatal care is the key to *staying* low-risk. And that midwives specialize in helping women stay healthy.

Now Sara reflects long and hard. She considers the pros and cons of each option, and the alternative birth center wins out. She also finds that she would definitely prefer a midwife. She shares her thoughts with her husband and together they come to a decision. They make an appointment with the midwife that Sara met earlier, and tell their physician of their change of plans.

Over the months that follow Sara discusses her birth plan with the midwife and her associates. She is very specific; does not want the baby taken away from her at all, and no "routine" testing done without her express permission. In fact, she plans to take the baby home several hours after the birth. Her midwives agree to support these choices.

Regarding her own experience, Sara wants freedom to move around during labor, and to take any position she wants. The midwives suggest exercises that will prepare her body to assume birthing postures. When she confesses to being chronically tense because of work, they teach her stretching and relaxation she can do on the job and help her take a long-term look at her work situation. She has also decided she wants no episiotomy when she delivers, so the midwives show her perineal massage. Although they say they seldom do episiotomies, she asks how they will prevent her from tearing, just to make sure.

During labor, Sara progresses normally until she reaches seven centimeters, at which point her progress stops. Her midwives suggest new positions, but nothing seems to help. Thinking back, Sara remembers reading that taking a shower with your husband can really help if you're stuck. So they decide to try it. The baby's head comes down a little, but her cervix stays the same. Discouraged, she starts to cry, and then looks deep inside to see if she's afraid or maybe holding back. What does she need to do to really let go??

Privacy—she remembers suddenly that she fantasized about laboring in private. She asks everyone to leave her for a little while—even her husband, though she asks him to stay right outside the door. Once alone, she feels more relaxed and tries first to connect with the baby. Then she concentrates on releasing her cervix and letting herself sink deeper into her sensation. Suddenly it's more intense, and she finds herself breathing faster. She calls her husband back. They labor together for an hour, and when the midwives check again she has only a rim of cervix left. Before long she is completely dilated and ready to push.

As delivery approaches, the midwives apply hot compresses to the perineum and Sara tunes in even more to her body's signals. The baby is born without a tear, and Sara and her husband are ecstatic with joy. As requested, the baby stays with them and is examined right there on their bed. The new family returns home just four hours after the birth.

Looking back on this example, see how Sara began by making herself knowledgeable. She collected information, talked with friends and went back to the books as necessary. She then proved herself decisive, although this required a major change in her original plans. Nevertheless, she communicated clearly to her care providers exactly what she wanted, down to the smallest detail. She also made certain they understood her requests, by finding out how they would meet her needs. And when obstacles arose in labor, she used her base of knowledge *and* her creativity to come up with a solution. She used the experience of pregnancy and birth to transcend herself, to grow.

Keep in mind that the above example is just one of many possible scenarios. As my own bias is towards home delivery, I deliberately avoided inserting this in the story. Perhaps you would prefer a home birth, or would honestly feel more comfortable in a traditional hospital situation. Whatever your plans, *take some time to fantasize and write out your ideal birth scenario, in as much detail as possible.* You may discover that you need to make some changes in your current situation if you expect to realize your dreams. Accomplishing for yourself all that Sara did is not impossible!

Now some specific guidelines for each basic type.

The Physical Type

When it comes to mental preparation, this woman's biggest problem is she tends to think she knows it all already! Or rather, that her body provides more tuned-in information regarding her needs than she can find in any book. There is certainly some truth in this attitude, but it has its limits. It will not help a woman handle unforeseen complications with any understanding, nor does it give her much of an advantage in negotiating treatment should difficulties arise.

The challenge for the physical type is to see that acquiring information need not negate physical intuition as her primary mode of operation. Factual information at her fingertips (or in the old back pocket) can only serve to strengthen her position in the event of need.

It is most important that she thoroughly study labor and birth, since checking a reference book once the process has begun is usually out of the question. Topics for study should include:

1) the mechanics of labor and delivery;

2) the whys and wherefores of various birthing positions and other coping techniques;

3) the causes and treatment of labor complications and emergencies;

4) routine tests for the baby, optional and mandatory;

5) the rudiments of breastfeeding.

Beyond her own understanding in these areas, she must also share plans and preferences with her birth attendants. Although I've mentioned this several times already, I cannot stress enough how important this is! Here is a list of common desires (you may add your own in the space provided):

1) privacy during labor and delivery (no parade of nurses, interns or medical students allowed);

2) birth in the labor bed (moving to the delivery room only in case of emergency);

3) dimmed lights at delivery, and no loud talking;

4) immediate rooming-in, with baby's exam at your bedside;

5) no routine tests for you or the baby without an explanation and your permission;

6) _____

_____

7) _____

_____

8) _____

_____

To give yourself every chance of getting what you want, ask to have a written copy of your requests attached to your chart. Frequently the physician does not arrive until you are well-advanced in labor, and you will be in no mood to argue with staff in the meantime. Your doctor may even be ill or performing surgery, thus a verbal agreement alone may not suffice.

It bears repeating that labor is not time to fight for what you want. To do so runs contrary to your need to be self-involved and vulnerable. *Make certain* that your partner understands your wishes, and his role in implementing them. This may require that he do a bit of study himself. Or if you prefer to have your partner with you strictly as a participant, then the responsibility to advocate your wishes can shift to a friend or other family member. Just be sure you have someone to look out for you.

If you are planning a home delivery, your wishes will probably be discussed and noted in your chart automatically. The same may be true of an ABC midwifery service, although if there are more than two providers on rotation, a list is a good idea.

Regarding the postpartum period, prepare in advance by reading a basic book on breastfeeding such as *Nursing Your Baby* by Karen Pryor or *The Womanly Art of Breastfeeding* by Le Leche League. It's true that breastfeeding is a spontaneous physical function, but it is definitely subject to emotional, environmental and nutritional factors. With a firm knowledge base established beforehand, you'll be free to nurse your baby without doubt or anxiety and will be much more likely to succeed if you know the pitfalls.

The Emotional Type

As has been stated already, the emotional woman's greatest challenge is to read broadly enough during pregnancy to develop her own perspective, rather than merely latching on to someone else's passionate viewpoint. This type tends to fanaticism, the only cure for which is deliberate exposure to diverse or even contradictory viewpoints until a distillation of knowledge can be acquired.

What are the most critical topics for research during pregnancy? This type often needs study in nearly every area:

1) nutrition for pregnancy;

2) prenatal exercise;

3) whys and wherefores of prenatal assessment;

4) sexuality and the childbearing cycle;

5) the mechanics of labor and delivery;

6) complications of labor and birth;

7) coping mechanisms for both normal and complicated birthing;

8) the basics of breastfeeding;

9) postpartum exercise and recovery;

10) newborn care.

There are several books of a general nature which can serve to cover most of these areas. *The Complete Book of Pregnancy and Birth,* by Shiela Kitzinger, has lovely illustrations and a sensitive, feminist perspective. Tracy Hotchner's *Pregnancy and Childbirth* is encyclopedic and a bit dry, but touches on nearly every subject. Rahima Baldwin's *Special Delivery* is particularly good for its clear and simple explanations of prenatal and labor complications. And my own book *Heart and Hands: A Midwife's Guide to Pregnancy and Birth* also covers these subjects in detail.

You should probably plan to purchase a book or two especially on baby care. A classic in the field is Penelope Leach's *Your Baby and Child.*

One of the most troublesome characteristics of the emotional type is her inability to communicate concretely her specific wishes and desires. She skirts the edges of these with allusion, and prefers to discuss her feelings about things rather than what she wants to *do* about them. Nevertheless, preferences regarding the birth and/or immediate care of the baby must be *spelled-out, written out, and shared with one's partner and birth attendants.* Check the list of possibilities on page 106, and once you've compiled your own, see that a copy is placed in your chart so that everyone who has anything to do with your labor or newborn will at least be aware of your wishes.

One more thing: do not neglect to read in the areas of breast-feeding and baby care while you are still pregnant! Pregnancy is the calm before the storm; the first few weeks of mothering are wild and crazy, partly due to hormone shifts and partl y to the soul-shaking change of becoming a parent. In other words, it's a tough time for rational thought and information gathering, particularly for those who tend to emotional extremes anyway.

The Mental Type

The main challenge for this type is to focus her information gathering with questions and concerns that are relevant to her *own situation*. She has a tendency to love information for its own sake and to lose herself in its pursuit. In fact, she may use information gathering as a way to avoid making decisions or taking action. This is the perpetual student, the type who never thinks she knows enough to make up her mind and who wants so much to be perfect that she may limit her experience (and her humanity).

If this is you, you need a framework for learning. Before studying, formulate a list of pertinent questions to serve as reference points. Say you want to read up on nutrition; note first any symptoms, special needs or health concerns you currently have. Perhaps you've been craving sugar and are suffering from leg cramps and late-afternoon depression. Write these things down on a note card and use it as a bookmarker; you can also use it to jot down page numbers if you choose. This way, you avoid being sidetracked by other fascinating information (you can always note subjects and page numbers for future research).

And once you have obtained information in your area of concern, make sure that you act on it! Outline a plan of action step-by-step, and definitely include a timetable.

Formulating and prioritizing questions for your care provider is another critical task. Just as the emotional type presumes others' emotional sensitivity, the mental woman tends to assume that all providers have a uniform standard of care and up-to-date knowledge base when in fact they do not. In other words, your midwife/physician may not be aware of the information and techniques you consider important, or may utilize practices contrary to your desires. The only way to find out is to ask, little by little, a few questions at each visit. Discussion will be easier and more to the point if your questions are specific; for example, rather than ask if the baby can stay with

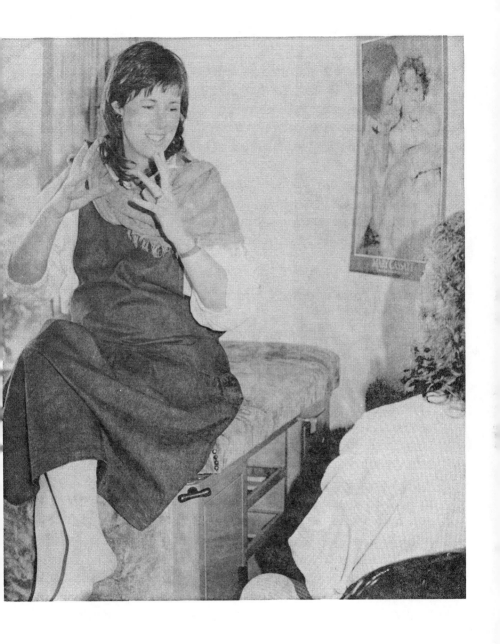

you continuously after the birth, find out what procedures are routine and whether or not they can be performed at your bedside.

Regarding postpartum research, it's a little hard to find focus when you've not yet had the baby. Try to obtain as much first-hand information as possible on breastfeeding and newborn care. Then let your reference books serve you at need (you'll be much more likely to stick to the subject at hand once you're busy with the baby!).

Do beware of reading child development or early education books before the birth. More on this in Chapter Nine, suffice for now that you maintain an open mind and wait for the nature and needs of your child to manifest with time.

If This Is Your Weakest Area

If this is your weakest area, you may never have learned to enjoy learning for its own sake. This is actually a common problem; our school system does little to encourage the development of independent thinking or the ability to do meaningful research. Think back to your days in first or second grade; do you remember not being allowed to turn the page of your reader or workbook until everyone else was finished? Or tediously having to listen to another student read aloud while your mind (and your eyes) were racing ahead? Or being stuck on some basic mathematical principle, with no one willing to take the time to help you understand on your own terms? Getting "points off" for having too many words in a composition, while the content went unnoticed? Not being allowed to choose your topic for a term paper, or having to follow such a strict format for a book report that you failed to convey the drama and excitement of your reading? This list is endless; I'm sure you could add a few frustrations of your own!

Because of this artificial and constricting learning style to which we were subjected, few of us learned genuine intellectual *discipline*. This includes being able to read long and complex works, to sort facts from dogma, formulate pertinent questions and do research. Only by developing some ability in these areas can we feel comfortable with the never-ending challenge of keeping informed. Of course it's easier to watch TV, read popular magazines or simplistic news articles to stay more or less abreast. But what about *personal* intellectual pursuits, the growth and development of our own interests, questions, train of thought?

One way to repair intellectual damage from school or media bombardment is to browse in a bookstore, scanning titles by subject area and whittling purchases down to the ones you know you'll read. But don't be afraid of a longer book with an intriguing table of contents, especially if it somehow connects with another of your primary interests. Try to keep yourself from routine TV watching; instead, jump in bed with a book at least a few nights a week. And get in the habit of keeping current reading by the phone for the inevitable periods you are put on hold, or take a book along when you go out, in case you must wait for an appointment.

Despite the fact that you are pregnant, don't feel that the only books you should read are those on birth or baby care. What you are attempting here is to give yourself a new lease on life intellectually. This means you get to read whatever interests you!

Once you begin reading for enjoyment, start keeping a notepad handy so you can jot down questions as they arise. It's unlikely you'll remember them later (you can always cross them out if they no longer seem pertinent). In terms of your reading on childbirth, these questions may be appropriate to ask your care provider or childbirth educator, and may serve to foster communication between you. *Don't be afraid to ask questions!* Again, our conditioning is that to profess ignorance is to appear the fool. But what could be more foolish than censoring one's own learning?

Take a chance now and then in social situations and raise

a topic for discussion that you consider intriguing. You may make new friends this way, or form intellectual liaisons that you'll find very satisfying. You will also encounter perspectives other than your own, which will suggest new areas for inquiry. Let your natural curiosity work for you, and don't be shy about showing your "smarts"!

Chapter 8

Developing A Support System

The need to develop a support system during pregnancy has been alluded to in every single chapter thus far. Why is this so important? Most societies provide support for new mothers automatically; at least this is true in nearly every country but the US and Canada. Here we must think in terms of *social preparation*, i.e., making the best use of what little society does offer to help ourselves learn to parent. And because this process is fairly universal, there are no basic type breakdowns in this chapter; it's for everyone.

First we must face the truth of what becoming a new mother means for most women in our culture. The need for recuperation is virtually unrecognized; a woman is expected to squeeze in what rest she can in the first couple days postpartum. Some women plan a longer stay in the hospital in hopes of a speedier recovery, but end up being so disturbed by routine monitoring of themselves and the baby that they leave severely sleep-deprived. And unless the new father is lucky enough to work

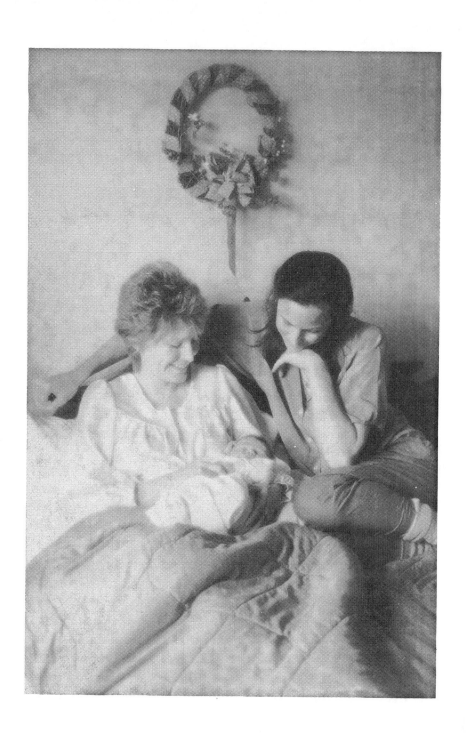

for a firm with an enlightened policy on paternal leave (or is just plain insistent) he too may suffer from the exhaustion and emotional strain of sleep deprivation. Thus parents are handicapped from the start, and desperately in need of support. If they are fortunate, their relatives may offer help with dinner for several nights or may run a few errands. But what if there is absolutely no one to fall back on?

Not to paint a grim picture, but the situation is nearly impossible. The new mother simply cannot manage housework, food shopping and preparation, her personal care and that of the baby plus breastfeeding without some assistance. As suggested earlier, she really should have at least four or five days *in bed* with no responsibilities except caring for the baby. Depending on the circumstances of the birth, this period of complete rest may need to be extended to ten days, or even more in the event of a Cesarean. This is not to say that she can't be up for meals, take some fresh air or chat with friends, but she cannot be expected to coordinate responsibilities and keep the household running smoothly. Therefore outside help is a *must*, be it from friends or paid assistants.

It's interesting to note that even though most women do something to prepare for birth and may even study up on complicated delivery or Caesarean, few make any preparation for the postpartum. I imagine many of you have already read discouraging descriptions like the one above, but have either thought, "I'll deal with it when the time comes," or, "That won't happen to me; I'm too strong, well-organized and resourceful." Why the brazen attitude, this refusal to look reality in the face?

The answer is quite simple: most of us can't, or more accurately *won't* believe that we could ever be so helpless or vulnerable. After all, we are *modern* women, proud of our executive abilities at home and in the workplace. We've learned to be tough, swift, in command. We gravitate towards images of birth that reinforce this identity; staying "on top" of contractions or "pushing" in second stage. Surrender and all it

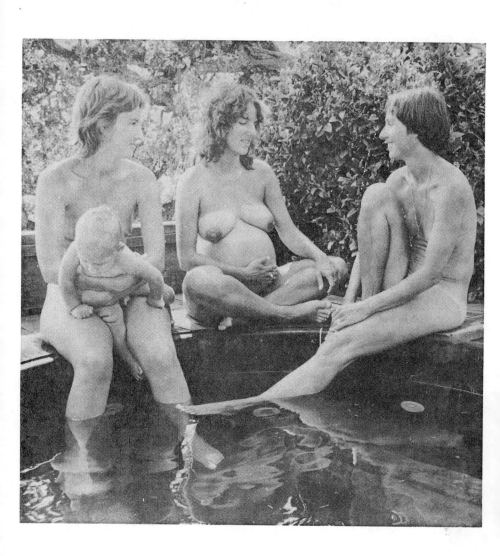

connotes doesn't really register; it means little more to us than unwinding at the end of a hard day's work. But like it or not, labor will call on us to let go, give in and be raw and exposed as never before. This would indeed be hard and horrible were it not for the empowerment in cooperating with the process, the sweetness of conscious birth and the incredible tenderness of the bonding period which are also our heritage as women.

Once more, *birth is an altered state,* and the first few weeks after an extension thereof. There is fragility, tenuousness, fatigue beyond telling, exhilaration, wild hope and genuine foresight, plus the physical challenges of recuperation and breastfeeding. This is a *transitional* phase, a time of flux, formulation and revolution, and just like transition during labor will lead to stability and adjustment if not tampered with.

But without adequate support, this phase may be curtailed or aborted. The reason why indigenous cultures place so much emphasis on this phase and essentially give the mother time-out is that group survival *depends* on her being fully recovered and thoroughly transformed to accept her new role. Most of us workaholic types have never really taken this sort of respite from our cultural obligations. Vacations help, but unless they are extended we may never really escape. Well, this is the time to do it; as frightening as it may seem at first, a *complete break* is necessary to reintegrate and be whole again.

It is hard to get around our cultural conditioning, but there are ways. Let's look at the tribal model a bit more closely for some guidelines.

In most of these cultures, preparation for birth and mothering is ongoing from the earliest years of childhood. Postpartum support is the natural result of intimate relationships developed over many years, in the context of extended family. Girls grow to womanhood witnessing the births of cousins, younger siblings, etc. and the deliveries of older sisters. Childcare is a shared responsibility, so that a girl is loved and mothered by many. Other aspects of lifestyle further serve to foster intimacy among the women, as they gather food and prepare it together, do the washing and handywork as a group. In these settings women often sing out spontaneously; they most definitely chat about the joys and struggles of their lives. Every major event in the female sexual cycle (menstruation, marriage/intercourse, childbirth and menopause) is marked by some sort of rite of passage, in affirmation that these are normal yet significant occurrences for the community. A young woman does not have to wonder what labor is like, whether she will be able to breastfeed or take care of a child because she has had intimate exposure to all of this by the time she comes of age.

Our task is to somehow acquire this intimate exposure, or the closest thing to it. It helps to visit places where mothers naturally congregate, like parks and playgrounds, for a little observation and candid conversation. Ask the women you meet about their birth experiences and what being a new mother is really like. Watch them with their babies and young children to see how they manage. If possible, take your partner along on the weekend so he can observe the fathers.

Organizations which focus on the early months of parenting or the needs of new mothers/fathers can be a tremendous help. Le Leche League, Int. has chapters throughout the US, and women are encouraged to attend meetings while still pregnant. Not only is there information on breastfeeding, but plenty of frank discussion of typical postpartum challenges and problems. And you will learn much simply by being in the same room with new mothers, through emotional osmosis.

Depending on how pregnant you are, you may still have time to take early-bird classes, either alone or with your partner. (It's nice to regroup with the same women/couples later on for your labor series; affords some social continuity.) And you must *definitely* take some kind of prenatal exercise class, be it yoga, aerobics or dance. Here is your best opportunity for making special friendships that may last into the early years of parenting. At the very least, you'll find someone to phone with minor questions about nursing, sleep schedules, diapering, etc. And think how nice it would be to be able to meet for tea while your babies play together, or to walk, shop and chat with your babies in their packs or strollers. Don't be too fussy about the intellectual quality of these relationships; you'll find much in common on a very basic level that should be quite sufficient for this time in your life.

Once you begin your labor series, you and your partner might try to cultivate a friendship with another couple in the class, particularly if they live nearby. Go out and get to know one another better; even if you haven't a lot in common you will in the very near future! Your babies needn't be more than a few weeks old before you might all take a drive in the country, or go to a drive-in movie together.

Even if you are planning a home delivery, check with your local hospital to see if they offer any classes on newborn care. Better yet, *offer to help a new mother for several hours with her routine chores.* If you don't know of anyone, ask your childbirth educator or care provider for suggestions. Of all my recommendations thus far, I consider this the most important! Especially if you have never been around babies before, why not learn basic diapering, bathing and coping skills in advance? Or if you and your partner happen to have friends who have recently had a baby, maybe they can give you a crash course.

At the very least, read a book on normal newborn behavior, appearance and care. You will be a lot less likely to have a nervous breakdown if you know in advance that the little white bumps that suddenly appear on your baby's face are not some horrible contagious disease but oil glands beginning to function, or that the little blue spots at the base of the spine are perfectly normal, etc. On the other hand, you should also be alerted to abnormal appearance and behavior, because unless your provider does routine home visits after the birth you will be very much on your own.

Sometimes it happens that friends will be delivering before you, and invite you to attend the birth. This would seem the ideal preparation and in many respects it is, but there are a few things to keep in mind. Your labor will probably be very different from what you witness, especially if this is your first baby and her second (or third). And if there are major complications you will definitely need some mental and emotional debriefing afterwards, via your provider or childbirth educator. But do offer your assistance postpartum; again, the osmotic effect will be most beneficial.

Birth films are a rather poor substitute for the real thing; they are generally so tightly edited that the true nature of labor (particularly hard labor) is not really portrayed. One of the best services ever available in my area was a monthly showing of birth videos—uncut (from transition on), uncensored and un-adorned (no music, special lighting, etc.). These were taken by the partner of a local midwife as a gift to the parents, and with their consent became a great service to the community. My own clients eagerly attended, and saw everything from "the screamer" (who wailed continuously until the baby was born) to "the madonna" (who sat beatifically without a sound until suddenly out popped the baby!). These had tremendous impact in that they imparted a sense of reality otherwise difficult to obtain.

And here's a suggestion that might seem a bit strange at first, but is actually recommended by the famous obstetrician Michel Odent and is common practice among tribal women. *Try singing with a group of pregnant friends,* or with women in your family. Singing gets you out of your head and into your heart, helps you shed your social mask (as you must during labor). It also opens various energy centers in your body, particularly those in your pelvis. Don't worry about being formal with this; three or four of you can sing along as you ride in the car, or in the quiet of someone's living room. Try it! It's a little awkward at first but you will grow to love it.

———————————————

Thus far, suggested activities have focused primarily on you and your partner. What about involving your relatives, your mother, sister(s) and the rest of your family?

Childbirth is undoubtedly one of the most transformative events for a family. If this is your first baby, you will be surprised at how your parents' view of you changes once you've given birth. And if this is their first grandchild, their own transformation will be even more surprising. Together you will enter a new phase of life wherein old tensions dissolve and new bonds are created. After all, you are a parent yourself now and you and your folks are basically in the same boat! You may find that you are actually eager to ask their advice, and may feel a great sense of relief as their focus shifts from you to your child. These changes are natural and fairly subtle, yet so very profound.

Your immediate family is an ideal source of postpartum support, but it must not be your *only* one. Although this is often the case in our culture, there are serious drawbacks to this arrangement. Family has by nature a somewhat limited scope, with inbred attitudes and beliefs generally made more extreme by stress. As there is almost no time in your life more stressful than the early weeks with a newborn, you will need the objectivity of those outside your family unit even if you must deliberately seek it out.

The bottom line in dealing with family members is to be *honest* and *clear* about what you do and do not want, what you can and cannot handle. *Be specific;* if Mom offers to help go ahead and ask her to take out the trash, scrub the toilet, whatever. And do be realistic about your emotional state at this time; your explosive and depressive tendencies, your outright limitations. It is not the end of the world if you have an angry outburst; your mother is old enough to understand and should be able to fend for herself.

Here is a sample list of typical postpartum needs. Your own list will depend on many variables, for example, it will be much more extensive if you have other children or are a single parent. At bare minimum, you will need:

1) dinner prepared for you at least five days (ideally ten).

2) someone to do your laundry for at least five days.

3) major housecleaning help once a week for six weeks.

4) food shopping for the first five days (if your partner can help with this, first few days is sufficient).

5) an errand-person on short notice for the first week (a must if your partner will be back at work).

6) one-on-one care for the first five days *minimum*. This depends on the circumstances of the birth; if in any way traumatic you'll need seven to ten days care. This can be your partner, but if he will be at work or you are single, you must find someone else.

There are many ways to deal with these requirements. Regarding the first, some women freeze enough meals to last a week, and stock the house as for an army. Nevertheless you'll still need fresh items, and someone to run for these. Often the father is willing, although he may be loathe to leave you and the baby for very long.

Help with the laundry is a must, particularly if you are washing diapers. Regarding the housecleaning, note the extended period recommended for assistance. Believe me, that's being conservative; ideally you would have someone weekly for the first year or more. The last thing you'll want to do with a few precious moments when the baby is finally asleep is to spend them mopping the floor!

Have you considered having your mother come and care for you? It may be hard to imagine now, but things will be different after the birth. Of course it depends on the size of your household and available space for guests. When I had my last baby, my husband and I were living with my two teenagers in a fairly small house. I had a rather long labor, so my mother offered to come and help out for a while. After thinking it over, she decided to stay at a nearby motel. She could afford it, and didn't mind as long as she could get to know her newest grandson. She was over every morning at about 8:00 (unless we requested otherwise) and left in the evening. Several nights she made dinner early and took the older kids back to her place to eat, so my husband and I could have some privacy. She did laundry, cleaning and was totally there for me emotionally. The length of her visit had been open-ended from the start; she ended up staying for two weeks. Looking back, this was a very precious time for us and one of the greatest gifts she has ever given me. But I must add that it took more than a little struggle through the years to enable us to be together this way.

Another tip for handling the stresses of the first few weeks is to fall back on a little personal indulgence when the going gets rough. Have a glass of wine, some special dessert or a gourmet dinner brought in, watch a movie on the VCR or take a drive to some special spot (with a little fast-food on the way). Treat yourself well and it will carry over to the baby. Particularly if the birth was difficult, consider hiring a bodyworker or masseuse to come every day for a week or so. It will make a tremendous difference in your energy level and your ability to cope. Choose a time when the baby is most likely to be content, and have someone available to take over just in case.

As the weeks and months go by, don't forget to make use of the various parenting services society does provide. Most every major metropolis has some sort of talk-line for parents at their wits' end (in San Francisco this is called the "warm line"). Subscribe to *Parents' Magazine, American Baby* or the more progressive *Mothering.* And check out a postnatal exercise class; these are often designed for both you and the baby (with childcare provided).

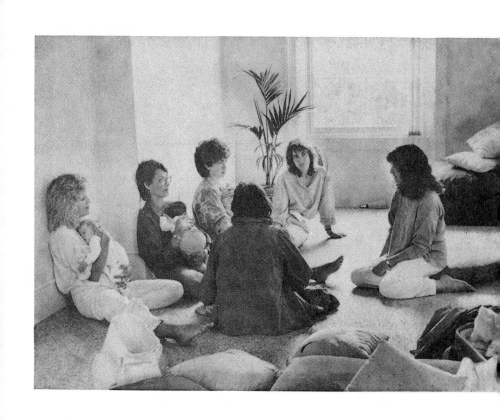

It's never too late to start a mothers group, even if you have to do it yourself. I'm reminded of my sister Carole who moved shortly before she had her baby; she knew no one in her area but walked right up to new mothers on the street or in the supermarket and introduced herself. Eventually she brought them all together for tea. They all appreciated the chance for adult companionship, and the opportunity to watch their babies interact and grow.

As your baby gets older, you might take him/her to a child development class at the local university for some play in an "enriched" setting. There are also programs such as *Gymboree*, which focuses on physical development, and the more interactive *Mommy and Me*. Whenever you feel the four walls closing in on you or the wait for Daddy to come home as endless, get outside for a walk or some activity, or give a good friend a call.

Although this is not a particularly popular position just now, I do think it's important for a mother to stay home with her baby as long as possible. I fully understand and respect the desire to work, but believe this must be viewed in terms of its impact on the child. When a woman absolutely *must* work for financial survival, that is a different story. But many women convince themselves that work is a necessity when in fact it's a choice.

Research has shown that the first three years are critical to a child's development, and that babies in particular need a one-on-one relationship. Even in the best of daycare situations your little one will cry uncomforted, be bored or frustrated without adequate attention to its needs. It is focused *continuity* of care that matters most, and even in a small group of five or six this is scarcely possible to provide.

Think also about the messages a child gets when placed in fulltime daycare. In effect, mother's work is more important than it is. Much has been said about quality vs. quantity of time, but to a child they may actually be the same thing! After all, children have no concept of waiting. It takes more than a little patience for an adult to wait an hour for an appointment; how can we expect a child to wait eight hours every day to see its mother? How can we hope to build trust under these circumstances?

I know these are hard questions but I think it's time we asked them, not only for the sake of our immediate families but for that of our society. Let's be *honest* about our young ones' needs, then consider how to meet them. We must do the best we can, but should never underestimate the intrinsic value of a mother's love and concern for her child.

To return to the tribal model once more, remember to teach your children well. Let siblings help with baby care, at the same time encouraging them to look after themselves. Write birth chronicles for each of your children; these will be important to them someday. Teach your children to respect their sexuality, and to honor and trust their bodies. If you have a daughter, share with her the wonders of being female as she grows to maturity. Set an example by relating to your women friends in an open, honest fashion. And help her cultivate her native intelligence; her instinct, intuition and personal discernment.

Chapter 9

Birth, Baby and Beyond

This closing chapter will explore the process of fulfillment through birth and parenting. We'll take an in-depth look at the experiences of several of our basic types, from early pregnancy to late postpartum. Here's a chance to take an overview, to see how all the phases fit together. See yourself in these tales if you will; they all have happy endings!

Jan has been mentioned once already; the karate expert who complained that her body was failing her around sixteen weeks of pregnancy. How did she fare in the end? With a bit of support and understanding, she began to find resources for coping with life besides physical strength. Slowly she began to let her guard down during prenatal visits and discuss some of the problems she was having with her mate. They were unmarried and as yet uncommitted, which had been alright before but was now beginning to bother her. The hardest thing for her to do while pregnant was to connect with other women. She needed the contact, but was afraid of the vulnerability and the emotions that might be unleashed. There was also an issue of trust, not something she was used to granting other women since her partner had not been faithful to her.

At first she berated her experience in exercise class as useless and annoying, but gradually acquired greater confidence in herself and her pregnant body. Meanwhile, her mate became increasingly involved in the pregnancy, more understanding and tender than ever before. She became more sensitive to the baby and began to educate herself responsibly for the birth. But she still kept her partner at arms-length, right up until labor.

Being true to form for a physical type, she was quite frustrated with the process of dilating. In fact, she complained mightily and made very slow progress. Her partner was at her side constantly, but she chose to ignore him and to focus on me and my assistant for support. This could take her only so far; when she had been stuck at 5 cms. for awhile we decided to leave her and Jack alone together. As we moved to the door she panicked, so we firmly directed her to stand with her arms around him and release her hips, knees and shoulders *and let him support her.* We stayed for a second to make sure she was OK, when the most amazing thing happened. She began to shake and struggle, then suddenly released as he gave her 100% care and attention. They labored this way throughout transition, she pushed beautifully and was totally thrilled to have a gorgeous baby boy.

Both parents bonded intensely with the baby, and began to take care of each other for the first time in the history of their relationship. Jan was fine for the first few days, but as the afterglow from the birth wore thin and her many acquaintances stopped coming by, she started to push herself. When I phoned her on day five she said she had been out shopping with the baby and was utterly exhausted.

I sensed that she was once more attempting to use physical strength to overcome emotional obstacles, so we had a heart-to-heart talk. Jack had asked her to marry him, she was elated but still uncertain. Her experience of vulnerability in labor had been very intense, and she wondered if she could let this into her life on a regular basis.

She obviously had some thinking to do, but in the meantime needed to focus on recuperating and getting to know the baby. I suggested she hold off on her decision until she and the baby were stable. Once again, permission to let go and take it easy made a big difference; she surrendered to a fuller experience of mothering.

When I saw her again nearly nine months later, she and Jack had married and were very happy. She was undeniably proud of her son's physical strength and development, but her relationship with him was tender and articulate. She spoke of how he had "opened up" her life and of how much fun she was having. From the armored and defensive woman who came to me initially, she had transformed into a full-faceted and relaxed human being (with an edge undeniably her own!).

Anna was a highly emotional woman, very in touch with her feelings and expressive of her inner-workings. She *loved* being pregnant, but suffered many physical symptoms (nausea, fatigue, leg cramps, constipation) that finally persuaded her to improve her diet and get some exercise. At first her nutritional research was woefully inadequate; she latched on to every new theory she encountered. But once she learned to look for salient points and observe her own body for feedback, she found a dietary plan that worked for her.

Her relationship with her partner was relatively new. They were married, and he seemed like a sensitive sort, but it was hard to tell because she so consistently interjected her own feelings and beliefs whenever we asked him a question. She would smile knowingly at us upon leaving, and he clearly felt ridiculous. Not surprisingly, their relationship began to suffer and we were treated to all the intimate details.

It was a good thing she had taken the trouble to get in shape for the birth because she had a very long labor. This was partly because she reacted to it from the start, instead of going about her normal activities as long as possible. In fact, my partner and I finally set an ultimatum, cleared out well-meaning friends and left her to labor alone with her husband. No more than an hour passed before she phoned, and we returned to find her labor well established.

She proceeded to dilate beautifully, but absolutely *hated* pushing. She whined and complained, tightening her legs and buttocks. Her husband kept trying to help her relax, encouraging her to let go, but she brushed him aside. We finally told her to quiet down and *listen* to what he had to say. We also used hot compresses and a mirror to help her focus, and at last she rallied herself for delivery. She gave birth to a beautiful baby girl.

In the days that followed she had no trouble relaxing with the baby, but was prone to episodes of borderline hysteria whenever the baby was especially fussy. She would blame herself, her partner, the environment, the culture, even the "planetary situation" for her little one's woes! This was very upsetting to her husband, and further undermined their communication. At this point we interceded on his behalf, and discussed the baby as a separate being with developmental impulses and responses *entirely independent* from any outside influences. She began to relax at this, and to see possibilities in relationship heretofore unexplored. We encouraged her to talk with other women she had met in prenatal classes, to find out what their babies were up to. Slowly she began to acknowledge her little girl's independence.

She and her partner continued to struggle and unfortunately separated six months after the birth. Nevertheless, she had definitely grown beyond her earlier self-absorption. She shared physical activity with her daughter in a spontaneous and joyous fashion, and although she still tended to chatter was clearly aware of the need to listen to her child.

A short time ago she called to tell me that she had remarried, was very happy and expecting again. When I asked her about her new relationship she said, "Well, I've changed a lot, I'm not so demanding and we really respect each other."

Another story of an emotional type comes to mind; this woman was the overly sensitive variety. She was so focused on her husband's struggles with becoming a parent that she found it hard to take care of herself. She was very sweet and caring, but rather weak and physically restrained. We urged her to exercise, to find support from other women for her *own* experience, her own ideas. And once she did so she provided a sense of stability for herself and her husband that reassured and delighted them both. They became closer and closer; she talked with him openly, candidly, even bawdily sometimes.

In labor they were as one, moving together with her contractions in a way both sensual and tender. She dilated very rapidly, but had trouble focusing on second stage until her husband sat behind her. Then they resumed working together and soon their son was born.

She continued to be relaxed but assertive throughout the postpartum period. The father was with the baby as much as possible. They truly co-parented their child, and remain happily married.

It seems that in these career-oriented times, examples of mental types abound. Kay first visited me by herself; she was thrilled to be pregnant but was definitely disturbed by her emotional and physical symptoms. She had done plenty of reading, but was out of shape and lacked vitality. And she continually rationalized her feelings.

When I met her husband I could understand why; he was a man with an answer for everything and the most rigid beliefs (though veiled by an open, flexible philosophy). Every time Kay tried to talk, Alex interrupted her with his own conclusions about what she was feeling.

Her physical side was the easiest place to start. She worked fulltime and had every intention of doing so right to the end, but identified swimming as something she could do in her spare time. She grew to love it, and to love her body because of it. Her circulation improved, her appetite leveled out and she became more confident in herself.

In addressing her emotional inhibitions, we simply suggested she come to prenatals alone now and then. Her husband was in the habit of coming with her, but we noticed that when it was "just us girls" she really let her hair down.

All of this effort proved critical to her success with labor. She had a large posterior baby, and a long labor that took every ounce of stamina she had developed (afterwards, she attributed it all to the swimming). Likewise, the stress and struggle of making progress necessitated repeated emotional release, and she had become so sure of herself in this regard that her husband could only cooperate.

Her biggest challenge was the postpartum period. She was more vulnerable than she had ever anticipated. Her husband (who had returned to work almost immediately) came up with an extensive lists of shoulds and shouldn'ts, regarding housework and the baby. Already he was attempting to impose a behavioral system on the child, and Kay was a nervous wreck from second-guessing her own instincts and spontaneous impulses. Even with nursing, she felt compelled to struggle for a schedule. We did our utmost to validate her natural abilities and encouraged her to get help with the house (as we had all along). But these were folks that for all their acquaintances were actually very isolated.

Time passed and we met again. As you might imagine, this couple was involved with the headiest notions of child-rearing, continually searching their baby for signs of "superior" development. But I observed that they both had a comfortable, relaxed physical demeanor with their daughter. Alex was clearly in love with little Jo, and Kay was much more inclined to let his comments and suggestions roll off her back. All in all, they seemed to have made a fairly smooth transition to parenting.

I had another client who came to me for both her first and second deliveries. The first time she was fanatically optimistic, depending on her extensive knowledge base to get her through labor. Although naturally fit (she had inherited great muscle tone) she was not particularly connected to her body, and definitely not in touch with her emotions. She talked a blue streak on almost any subject, as if to prevent awkward or revealing silences.

One of her greatest assets was her mate, who was very sensitive and concerned for her welfare. Still, it was obvious that they had settled into a pattern wherein she was the rational voice; a pattern that was rapidly becoming outmoded because of pregnancy.

Once in labor, this woman quickly learned that relaxation meant something altogether different than what she had bargained for, and that she'd have to go farther in bearing sensation than she ever imagined. She panicked at home, wanted nothing more than to go to the hospital for pain relief. Later she confided that all the time I was trying to help by encouraging her to relax, she secretly wanted to kill me! Her postpartum was tempestuous; the birth had so altered her self-image and relationship with her husband that she was quite disoriented.

When she returned to me pregnant with her second child, I was more than a little uncertain about assisting her. But it soon became obvious that she had mellowed through the experience of parenting, and that she and her partner were on more equitable terms. As it turned out she had a fast and fairly easy labor—a great triumph for her and a boon to the entire family.

And how did she mother her children? Her first was so clever, wiley and willful that the struggle between them was non-stop. But the second child was more easy-going, and she surrendered to a more instinctive approach with both.

Now let's use these stories to extrapolate some basic guidelines for baby and childcare. Once more, these suggestions will be presented according to basic type.

The Physical Type

When it comes to baby care, the physical type may be a bit brazen about her baby's needs and may find herself emotionally shutting down whenever the baby cries. She may feel pushed or angered by its constant demands, or may fear she will spoil it if she gives in to its every call.

Rest assured, there is no such thing as too much loving for a baby! Consider how totally secure your little one was in utero; all its needs completely met with never a delay. Naturally it needs constant reassurance in the early weeks, but eventually this gives way to some semblance of stability as fear and uncertainty subside.

Not surprisingly, the physical type of woman often relies on *stimulation* to keep her baby happy. Baby swings, bouncy seats, etc. are useful to a point; many babies derive great comfort from rhythmic movement. But babies also need to be calmed and *quieted* through sensitive touch and careful handling, especially in the early weeks. If the baby is crying and nothing at all seems to work, let the baby feel the warmth of your body and hear the love in your voice as you walk or gently rock it.

You may have to calm *yourself* down considerably in order to do this!

Little babies are very vulnerable to the intensity of the outside world; they dislike bright lights, loud noises, strange odors, crowds. I remember trying to take my son to a department store when he was six weeks old (I was looking for a nursing bra—should have gotten it before!). This was one of our first indoor outings; we had already been on numerous drives and walks. After about two seconds on the escalator, he let out a blood-curdling scream that sent me running for the nearest exit. It wasn't until he was about nine months old that environments like this were at all acceptable to him.

The greatest challenge for the physical type is to honor the sensitivity and individuality of her child, rather than simply packing it along through her own whirlwind of activities. It is very important to *provide consistency* by respecting your little one's schedule: nap times, meal times, indoor and outdoor play times. Any experienced mother will tell you what her evening is like if her child misses his/her afternoon nap! Babies are simply creatures of habit; they look to their parents to bring order out of a seemingly chaotic world.

Following a schedule may sound boring to you, but try to innovate *within* structure. This is good discipline for anyone, and essential for getting things accomplished. Perhaps you are beginning to see what I meant earlier when I said that babies force us to change and grow. Besides, you can always get out for a little free-flow on your own time now and then. In fact, make it a point to do so!

Learn about the stages of child development during the first few years. You may be surprised to find that there are definite phases of stability and chaos, all contributing to overall growth. Learn which toys your baby is apt to enjoy and why, and how verbal skills develop.

A general rule of thumb when caring for a little one is to *think small*, focusing on the process, rather than the idea or result. For example, if your child seems bored, temperamental or frenetic, focus on *one toy* (like a little animal) and give it life, speech, movement, etc. This will appeal to your child's imagination and will reunite scattered energies.

Take care to avoid accidents if your baby does become over-stimulated or overtired. For example, a child just learning to walk will tend to stumble and fall as the day progresses, especially if upset.

And what is the pay-off for all this attention and nurturing? If your baby is happy, the two of you will be able to get out more and gradually share activities. The more trustworthy and reliable you are, the more confident and independent your little one will become. *You will find freedom and mobility without having to abandon your child.*

The Emotional Type

Unlike her physically-oriented sister, the emotional woman tends to stay home more with the baby, which is basically good. But she also tends to float through the day and lose track of time, which is hard on her child. Routine events, at predictable times, are critical punctuation in an otherwise unstructured day. This means being aware of naps times, meal times, quiet hour, etc. If there is one thing little ones do not tolerate well, it is waiting! This includes waiting with you in line, waiting while you talk on the phone or chat with a friend, etc.

Take a moment to consider why this is so. When newly born, a baby cries at the slightest frustration because up until now all its needs have been completely met. It has been warm, nourished and rocked in utero, all the while comforted by the sounds of your heartbeat and voice. It has never been cold, hungry or lonely. There is no way it can know that you are nearby in the next room, or that you will nurse it "as soon as you get off the phone." You cannot teach a baby tolerance for frustration by forcing the issue! But if you are reliable and dependable in meeting its needs, it will soon feel secure enough to be patient—for a moment or two! Gradually this period of time will lengthen, as long as you don't abuse its trust with your own self-indulgence. This is why you need time away from the baby, to give you a chance to satisfy your more personal needs.

Another challenge for the emotional type is to provide *focused stimulation*. This is not important at first, since all a newborn really needs is tender loving care. But as your baby grows, he/she will crave creative play, new faces, outings appropriate for its age and development. This requires that you overcome your own inertia and get out more, try new things. But you must also appreciate the phases of growth your little one is going through. Read a book on child development, making sure you select one with lots of information on the first year.

Getting together with other mothers and babies will help you acquire perspective. It is always a bit of a shock to discover that a baby the same age as yours makes almost the same sounds, movements, faces. You are so sure your baby is utterly unique! But then, it can be enlightening to hear what other mothers are doing to handle common problems. Plus, here is your chance to relax and chat while your baby plays with the others.

Sometimes emotional women fret and worry about letting their baby mingle, particularly if they have high ideals about upbringing. The best idea is to *see what the baby likes*. Some are social beings through and through, while others are little homebodies. Remember that your child is an individual, and don't project your beliefs on him/her.

Again, it is critical to appreciate the phases your child goes through so you don't get too tangled up in them yourself. Otherwise you might project feelings of displeasure, anxiety, or distress *without even knowing it*, making your child feel guilty or unloved. Emotional women tend to underestimate their power in this regard. Emotional intensity is a gift, but it can definitely be abused unless it is tempered with awareness and intelligence.

Understanding what is going on with the baby will also help to ease your own reactions. If you feel guilt or anger and keep holding back, you may explode in a violent outburst. Don't let this happen! Try talking to friends or your pediatrician, and learn to detach enough so your baby can grow with integrity. This may mean temper tantrums, contrariness or sullenness at times, but these are parts of life. If you can stay rational, you will be a source of strength when your little one is upset or confused.

The Mental Type

The mentally oriented woman remains true to form by trying to get her baby on a schedule. Schedules are not all bad; as mentioned earlier, babies need structure and order in their days. But there is a difference between imposing a schedule and following the baby's own.

In the early weeks particularly there is very little that remains constant from day to day; even nursing frequency will vary somewhat. The best approach is to follow the baby's lead and devote yourself to meeting his/her needs. There really is no way around this anyhow, unless you want a very fussy infant on your hands! In time, by about six months or so, regular napping and nursing rhythms are established. Then just when you think you've got it down, everything changes again. But at least nursings are less frequent and sleep times longer and more reliable.

Along these lines, you'll discover that child development books go only so far. More than any other type, the mental woman expects her child to grow by the book, to be at (or preferably above) developmental norms. But your baby is an individual, and may greatly excel in one regard while being rather slow in another. Besides, it is quite probable that your child is not the same type as you, which will make its orientation to life completely different from yours. If you are busy searching for signs of "reading readiness" while overlooking your baby's superior motor skills, chances are you will both feel very frustrated.

At this point I feel compelled to mention the growing concern among child development experts regarding the big push for early reading/academic skills. In contrast is the Waldorf system, which maintains that the early years should be structured entirely around imaginative play. They cite a critical turning point from inner world/family to outer world/society around age seven, at which time children with no previous reading experience are soon at or above the level of those who have been reading all along. As always, I think it best to tune in to the nature of your child, rather than imposing any system or philosophy. This does require a certain surrender to the task of parenting, much like that required during labor. The result may be just as surprising; an unexpected feeling of being in control, abreast, in harmony with the process.

This largely depends on your willingness to learn from your child. The mentally oriented woman tends to be so outwardly focused that she sees her child as a blank slate, needing to be trained and instructed in everything. But you will be surprised at how much your baby already knows, if you just slow down and pay attention. Babies are creatures of great sensate capacity, continually reflecting the truth of the world around them. Uncorrupted by philosophy or rational thought, they reflect how the ways of the world impact on basic human sensitivity. It is a privilege to be thus reawakened and revitalized by a child. Make no mistake, our children are our teachers.

One more thing: beware of overprotecting your little one from physical experimentation. A colleague recently recounted a morning spent with a new mother of the mental persuasion. She noticed that every time the baby came close to discovery through exploring its physical boundaries, the mother automatically lifted and moved it to another location. We must allow our children to take some risks in order to grow strong and confident. One way to help your little one feel comfortable with

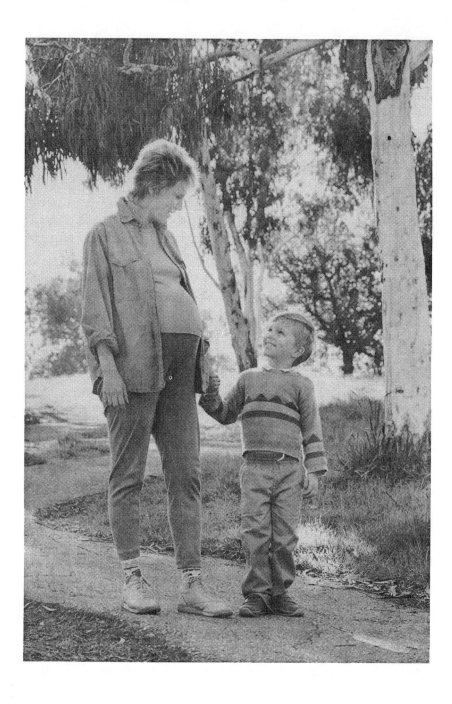

his/her body (and to get you into yours a bit more too) is to roughhouse, do some tickling and rolling around on the rug, or play some silly little nonsense games like peek-a-boo or hide-and-seek. Babies also love rhythmic activities (harking back to the womb, the sound of your heartbeat) and love hearing you sing and croon in a rhythmic fashion. Later, clapping games are lots of fun.

And take the time to enjoy the physical pleasure of your child. Hold your baby close, be skin-to-skin, and let feeling flow from your body. Go ahead and speak your love! What a difference this can make in a tense moment!

The bottom line in all of this is to work creatively with your assets and liabilities, at the same time respecting those of your child. The process of parenting is a lot like dancing; each of your children (if you have more than one) will be an altogether different partner, and you'll have to adapt your style to theirs. Not sacrifice or change, but *adapt*. Were this approach extended to our professional relationships, or our international relations country-to-country, we might actually build global community. Despite its seeming lack of significance in this culture, the family is indeed the cornerstone of society, *humane* society.

Your efforts to raise your child to be free, to respect him/herself and others, to perceive the world with tolerance and understanding therefore make a tremendous difference. The work you do while pregnant is a step in the right direction. Lift your illusions about yourself, develop a sense of humor about your foibles, and you will be wise and beneficent with your little one. *What else in life can so evoke our latent abilities, and so infuse the challenge of development with love as the process of parenting?* Have faith in this process and in yourself. We are all in this together!

0681 1490